MCQs in the Basic Sciences for the MRCP Part 1

MCQs in the Basic Sciences for the MRCP Part 1

J. S. Elborn MD, MRCP
Consultant Physician, Belfast City Hospital, Belfast

R. H. Evans MB BCh, MRCP
Registrar in Infectious Diseases, University Hospital of Wales, Cardiff

CHAPMAN & HALL MEDICAL
London · Weinheim · New York · Tokyo · Melbourne · Madras

Published by Chapman & Hall, 2–6 Boundary Row, London SE1 8HN, UK

Chapman & Hall, 2–6 Boundary Row, London SE1 8HN, UK

Chapman & Hall GmbH, Pappelallee 3, 69469 Weinheim, Germany

Chapman & Hall USA, 115 Fifth Avenue, New York NY 10003, USA

Chapman & Hall Japan, ITP Japan, Kyowa Building, 3F, 2-2-1, Hirakawacho, Chiyoda-ku, Tokyo 102, Japan

Chapman & Hall Australia, 102 Dodds Street, South Melbourne, Victoria 3205, Australia

Chapman & Hall India, R. Seshadri, 32 Second Main Road, CIT East, Madras 600 035, India

First edition 1998

Typeset in 9.5/11pt Times by Acorn Bookwork, Salisbury, Wiltshire

Printed in Great Britain at St Edmundsbury Press, Bury St Edmunds, Suffolk

ISBN 0 412 79280 X

A catalogue record for this book is available from the British Library

Library of Congress Catalog Card Number: 97–75070

∞ Printed on permanent acid-free text paper manufactured in accordance with ANSI/NISO Z39.48–1992 and ANSI/NISO Z39.48–1984 (Permanence of Paper)

Contents

Foreword

The foundation on which we base the practice of Medicine is provided by an understanding of basic biomedical sciences. The last twenty years have seen an explosion of interest in the field, prompted by the advances in molecular biology, but now encompassing all aspects of biomedical research. These advances have resulted in a greater understanding of pathogenesis and are leading to improved diagnosis and logical therapy, as well as opening up novel therapeutic approaches by applying the 'new biology'.

The Royal Colleges have recognized this important endeavour, and the increasing importance of being able to apply its knowledge-base into clinical practice, by incorporating questions into the written parts of professional examinations. However, the hard-pressed candidate, often having to find time to study for these examinations in the middle of busy junior hospital appointments, is faced with a bewildering plethora of facts. How to sieve the important from the minor when, after all, only a small fragment can be examined in the format of an MCQ can be a fruitless and frustrating task.

The authors of this interesting series of test questions have sought to identify some of the major topics covering most clinical subspecialties, and provide a useful commentary to guide the student. By its orientation, this book is directed at those studying for MRCP Part 1 – either in Medicine or Paediatrics – although it may be useful for anaesthetic and surgical candidates as well. It will prove useful to identify the gaps in a student's knowledge, set them on the path to understand the reasons for common errors in this type of question, as well as directing their further study. Perhaps most importantly of all, it will give them the confidence to tackle the 'basic' questions in the MRCP Part 1 examination, which, after all, are no more straightforward or difficult than other aspects of the paper.

L.K. Borysiewicz
Professor of Medicine
University of Wales College of Medicine, Cardiff, UK

Introduction

There has been an enormous expansion in biomedical science research during the past decade. The impact of molecular biology on the understanding of pathophysiology, diagnosis and management of disease is increasing significantly year by year. The multiple choice question examination for the MRCP Part 1 diploma reflects this change by having an increasing number of questions which relate to basic medical science. In addition to anatomy, physiology, biochemistry and pharmacology, molecular sciences are increasingly being asked about in this and other postgraduate diplomas. The areas covered by biomedical science are enormous in scope and it is very difficult for any individual to cover all topics.

This book attempts to cover some of the subjects which might result in questions in the MRCP Part 1 exam and in other postgraduate diplomas. We have tried to cover basic sciences such as molecular biology, genetics, statistics and epidemiology and have systematically gone through the major organ systems and developed questions based on the anatomy, physiology, biochemistry, pharmacology and molecular biology of diseases relating to these organ systems. We have not comprehensively covered all of the potential areas from which questions could be selected but we hope that this book is helpful in preparation for the MCQ examination for the MRCP. The practice of completing MCQs and using them as a stimulus to further reading is an efficient way of preparing for the MRCP Part 1 examination. Some suggestions for further reading are listed at the end of each chapter and these include both textbooks and papers. We would particularly recommend students to read recent reviews in the *Lancet*, *Nature*, *Medicine*, *The New England Journal of Medicine* and *The British Medical Journal* for updates on developments in science.

A number of these questions will soon be superseded by further developments in research and we ask the reader to be aware of this. There are also likely to be some answers with which the reader disagrees and we welcome any comments regarding these.

1 Basic molecular and cell biology

QUESTIONS

1.1 G proteins:
(a) bind ATP.
(b) are composed of three sub-units.
(c) link cell surface receptors to secondary messenger pathways.
(d) are commonly mutated in patients with acromegaly.
(e) are unaffected by *Vibrio cholerae* toxin.

1.2 Regarding the eukaryotic cell cycle:
(a) cell division occurs in the G_0 phase.
(b) cells in the G_1 phase have half the amount of DNA as those in the G_2 phase.
(c) the G_2 stage of interphase immediately precedes mitosis.
(d) DNA replication is restricted to the S phase.
(e) vincristine is only effective in the M phase.

1.3 *ras* oncogenes
(a) are mutated proto-oncogenes.
(b) are derived from viral nucleic acid.
(c) encode transmembrane growth factor receptors.
(d) are the most frequently observed oncogenes in human tumours.
(e) are activated in most cases of pancreatic adenocarcinoma.

1.4 The following statements are correct:
(a) the technique of Northern blotting utilizes labelled DNA probes to detect RNA.
(b) DNA fragments can be analysed by Southern blotting.
(c) Eastern blotting can detect sequence differences in DNA fragments using restriction enzymes.
(d) Western blotting may be used to identify a specific protein in a mixture of proteins.
(e) the polymerase chain reaction (PCR) can be used to amplify DNA but not RNA.

1.5 The following statements regarding the polymerase chain reaction (PCR) are correct:
(a) the technique uses the enzyme *Taq* DNA polymerase.
(b) the temperature of the reaction should not exceed $37°C$.

(c) primers only anneal to their complementary DNA sequence.
(d) the number of DNA copies increases tenfold after each cycle.
(e) PCR is not sufficiently sensitive for use in antenatal screening of genetic diseases.

1.6 Regulatory growth factors:
(a) are glycoproteins.
(b) characteristically exert paracrine effects.
(c) bind to receptors in the nuclear membrane of the cell.
(d) have close structural homology with steroid hormones.
(e) can be synthesized using recombinant DNA techniques.

1.7 The following statements regarding clotting factor V are correct:
(a) the gene for factor V is located on chromosome 1.
(b) factor Va is a natural anticoagulant.
(c) factor V Leiden occurs due to a single amino acid substitution in the factor V molecule.
(d) factor V Leiden is resistant to proteolysis by activated protein C.
(e) patients with factor V Leiden have an increased risk of venous thromboembolism.

1.8 Nitric oxide:
(a) is a free radical.
(b) is a neurotransmitter.
(c) inhibits platelet aggregation.
(d) has cytotoxic properties.
(e) causes systemic hypotension.

1.9 Nitric oxide synthases (NOSs):
(a) use L-arginine as a substrate.
(b) exist in three isoforms.
(c) are all calcium-independent.
(d) are confined to the vascular endothelium.
(e) may be induced by tumour necrosis factor alpha (TNFα).

1.10 The following statements are true:
(a) the gene for apolipoprotein E is located on chromosome 21.
(b) the apolipoprotein $\varepsilon 4$ allele is associated with an increased risk of developing Alzheimer's disease.
(c) the apolipoprotein $\varepsilon 2$ allele is associated with a reduced risk of Alzheimer's disease.

(d) familial Alzheimer's disease has been linked to mutations in chromosome 14.
(e) autosomal dominant familial Alzheimer's disease accounts for over 50% of all cases.

1.11 Tumour necrosis factor (TNF):
(a) is synthesized by mast cells.
(b) stimulates the satiety centre in the brain.
(c) enhances the microbicidal activity of phagocytes.
(d) upregulates adhesion molecules on endothelial cells.
(e) is responsible for the syndrome of Gram-negative endotoxic shock.

1.12 Interleukins:
(a) are synthesized mainly by macrophages.
(b) are proteins.
(c) are all pro-inflammatory.
(d) may induce fever.
(e) act as haemopoietic growth factors.

1.13 Apoptosis:
(a) is the principal mode of cell death in ischaemic necrosis.
(b) is characteristically associated with cell lysis.
(c) is caused by failure of the ionic pumps of the plasma membrane.
(d) does not provoke an inflammatory response.
(e) is inhibited by the oncogene *bcl-2*.

1.14 Anti-sense oligonucleotides:
(a) are sections of RNA.
(b) penetrate the cell membrane efficiently.
(c) block RNA processing.
(d) replace defective tumour suppressor genes.
(e) can be used to target viral nucleic acid.

1.15 Prion proteins:
(a) are viruses.
(b) are derivatives of normal cell membrane proteins.
(c) are not denatured by ionizing radiation.
(d) cause Huntington's disease.
(e) can be transmitted by corneal grafts.

1.16 Trinucleotide repeat diseases:
(a) are all inherited in an autosomal dominant manner.
(b) exhibit anticipation.
(c) exhibit genetic imprinting.
(d) include the fragile X syndrome.
(e) include Li Fraumeni syndrome.

1.17 The p53 protein:
(a) is a transcription factor.
(b) occurs only in malignant cells.
(c) arrests the cell cycle at the G_1 phase.
(d) synthesis is stimulated by ionizing radiation.
(e) is absent in the Li Fraumeni syndrome.

1.18 Inflammatory mediators derived from arachidonic acid include:
(a) histamine.
(b) leukotrienes.
(c) thromboxane A_2.
(d) prostaglandin I_2 (prostacyclin).
(e) bradykinin.

1.19 The following statements are true:
(a) prostaglandin $F_{2\alpha}$ is synthesized via the lipoxygenase pathway.
(b) prostaglandin I_2 is a bronchodilator.
(c) thromboxane A_2 is a vasoconstrictor.
(d) leukotrienes are more potent bronchoconstrictors than histamine.
(e) cyclo-oxygenase is directly inhibited by salicyclic acid.

1.20 Bradykinin:
(a) is a peptide.
(b) is a vasoconstrictor.
(c) activates phospholipase A_2.
(d) causes smooth muscle spasm.
(e) is inactivated by angiotensin-converting enzyme in the lung.

1.21 Interleukin-1 (IL-1)
(a) is synthesized predominantly by macrophages.
(b) synthesis is stimulated by tumour necrosis factor (TNF).
(c) stimulates proliferation of fibroblasts.
(d) induces the expression of endothelial cell adhesion molecules.
(e) is implicated in the pathogenesis of rheumatoid arthritis.

1.22 Cell adhesion molecules responsible for binding leucocytes to endothelium include:
(a) ICAM-1.
(b) E-selectin.
(c) β_2 integrin.
(d) complement receptor 3 (CR3).
(e) RANTES.

1.23 Recognized neutrophil chemotactic molecules include:
(a) interleukin-8 (IL-8).
(b) C5a.
(c) leukotriene B4.
(d) RANTES.
(e) interleukin-5 (IL-5).

1.24 Natural killer (NK) cells:
(a) are lymphocytes.
(b) express the T cell receptor (TCR).
(c) have receptors for the Fc fragment of IgG.
(d) have a role in lysing virus-infected cells.
(e) recognize and kill tumour cells.

1.25 Diseases caused by abnormalities in mitochondrial DNA include:
(a) Becker muscular dystrophy.
(b) Leber's hereditary optic atrophy.
(c) Leigh disease.
(d) myoclonic epilepsy and red ragged fibres (MERRF).
(e) familial progressive external ophthalmoplegia syndrome.

ANSWERS

1.1 (a) F (b) T (c) T (d) T (e) F
G proteins are so-named because of their ability to bind the guanine nucleotides GTP and GDP. G proteins are composed of α, β, and γ sub-units, and essentially function as on–off switches for cell signalling. Receptors coupled to one or more G proteins include those for catecholamines, thyrotropin-releasing hormone (TRH), gonadotrophin releasing hormone (GnRH), and β-adrenergic receptors.

Increased G protein activity is seen in 40% of patients with acromegaly secondary to pituitary somatotroph tumours, the thyroid autonomy syndrome, McCune–Albright syndrome, ovarian, adrenal and thyroid tumours, and *Vibrio cholerae* infection (cholera).

Reduced G protein activity is seen in pseudohypoparathyroidism (Albright's hereditary osteodystrophy).

1.2 (a) F (b) T (c) T (d) T (e) T

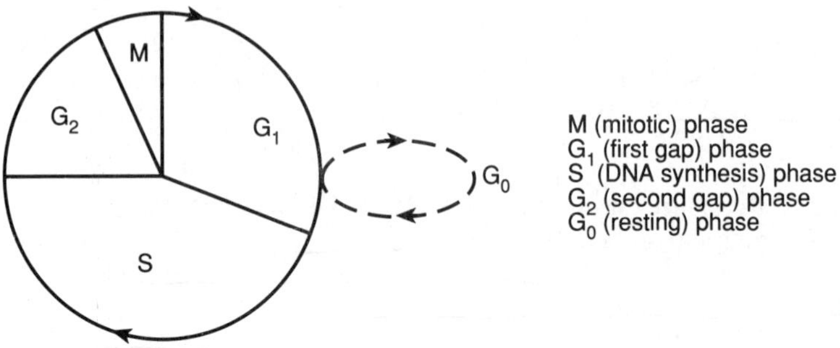

Figure 1.1 The cell cycle.

A cell in the G_1 phase (before DNA synthesis) has half the amount of DNA as a cell in the G_2 phase. The phases G_1, S and G_2 are collectively known as the interphase, i.e. the period between mitoses. Many cells suspend the cell cycle after dividing and before DNA synthesis – these are said to be resting in the G_0 phase (Figure 1.1).

Many anti-cancer drugs are only effective during parts of the cell cycle. These are termed phase-specific drugs. Drugs which are S-phase-specific include cytarabine (inhibits DNA polymerase), methotrexate (inhibits dihydrofolate reductase), fluorouracil (inhibits thymidylate synthetase), mercaptopurine and thioguanine (block purine ring synthesis). The vinca alkaloids vincristine and vinblastine inhibit mitosis by binding the protein tubulin, essential for spindle formation, and are therefore M phase-specific.

1.3 (a) T (b) F (c) F (d) T (e) T
Most oncogenes are derived from normal cellular genes called proto-oncogenes, whose products act along normal growth-controlling pathways. Proto-oncogenes and oncogenes encode several types of molecule, including growth factors, growth factor receptors, cytoplasmic enzymes, intracellular signal transducers and transcription factors. Oncoproteins, the protein products encoded by oncogenes, can transform cells to malignancy.

The largest class of oncogenes are those whose proto-oncogenes encode proteins which transmit signals from a cell surface receptor to an intracellular target (signal transduction). The *ras* proteins are guanine nucleoside-binding proteins with GTPase activity, and have some structural homology with G proteins. They are located on the inner surface of the plasma membrane. A single amino acid substitution is sufficient to change the *ras* proto-oncogene into an oncogene. Mutant *ras* is the commonest activated oncogene in human tumours – a specific mutation (K-*ras*) is seen in 90–95% of cases of pancreatic adenocarcinoma. Other malignancies associated with mutant *ras* include colonic adenocarcinoma, thyroid carcinoma and acute myeloid leukaemia.

1.4 (a) T (b) T (c) F (d) T (e) F
Immunoblotting techniques can detect DNA, RNA or proteins. Southern blotting takes its name from Edward Southern, who devised the technique, and allows detection of specific sequences of DNA in a complex mixture of DNA. DNA is cleaved into restriction fragments which are then separated by gel electrophoresis and 'blotted' onto a nitrocellulose membrane; a radioactive DNA probe is used to detect the position of the fragment of interest. Northern blotting uses a similar technique to detect RNA using a labelled DNA probe. Western blotting is used to detect a specific protein in a mixture of proteins using gel electrophoresis, nitrocellulose blotting, and a specific antibody to the target protein. Eastern blotting does not exist.

Both DNA and RNA can be studied by PCR, but RNA must first be translated into complementary DNA (cDNA) using the viral reverse transcriptase enzyme.

1.5 (a) T (b) F) (c) T (d) F (e) F
Reagents required for PCR:

1. DNA sample;
2. two single-stranded oligonucleotide primers (complementary to a specific sequence of interest);
3. heat-stable *Taq* DNA polymerase derived from *Thermus aquaticus* – an organism which naturally inhabits hot-water springs; and
4. the four nucleotides – adenine, guanine, thymine and cytosine.

The polymerase chain reaction has three principal steps: high-temperature DNA strand separation; low-temperature primer binding; and intermediate-temperature DNA synthesis. The cycle begins at 94°C to split the double-stranded DNA into two single strands. The temperature is then lowered to 55°C to allow the primers to bind (anneal) to the section of interest in the gene. The temperature rises to 72°C for optimal DNA synthesis, and a new double strand of DNA is synthesized by the *Taq* DNA polymerase. The cycle is then repeated, with the DNA templates produced in the first round acting as templates for the second round, such that after each cycle the number of copies is doubled. PCR is a rapid, specific and highly sensitive technique. The numerous applications of the PCR include diagnosis of infectious diseases, diagnostic oncology, carrier screening, antenatal screening, tissue typing and forensic medicine.

1.6 (a) T) (b) T (c) F (d) F (e) T

Peptide regulatory growth factors (haemopoietic growth factors, epidermal growth factor, etc.) act principally by paracrine secretion. Peptide growth factors are water-soluble molecules which bind to specific membrane-bound receptors which convert the primary message into a secondary intracellular message which stimulates mitosis. Steroids are lipid-soluble hormones which diffuse across the plasma membrane and interact with intracellular receptors.

Clinical uses of growth factors synthesized by recombinant DNA techniques include granulocyte-colony stimulating factor (G-CSF), used to stimulate recovery from neutropenia, epidermal growth factor (EGF), used to promote mucosal regeneration in infantile necrotizing enterocolitis; and erythropoietin (Epo), used to correct the anaemia associated with end-stage chronic renal failure.

1.7 (a) T (b) F (c) T (d) T (e) T

The gene for factor V is located on the long arm of chromosome 1. Factor V Leiden occurs because of a point mutation in the factor V gene (a glutamine for arginine substitution at position 506), and results in resistance to activated protein C (APC). APC is a natural anticoagulant which cleaves Va and VIIIa, thereby inhibiting the conversion of X to Xa and prothrombin to thrombin.

Venous thromboembolism is associated with defects in a number of molecules, including antithrombin III, protein C, protein S, plasminogen and fibrinogen. However, defects or deficiencies of these molecules only occur in 5–10% of patients with recurrent deep venous thromboses (DVT). The recently described mutation in the factor V molecule – designated factor V Leiden - has been shown in approximately 20% of patients with DVT.

1.8 (a) T (b) T (c) T (d) T (e) T

Nitric oxide (NO; endothelium-derived relaxing factor, EDRF) is synthesized from L-arginine and oxygen by the enzyme nitric oxide synthase. NO is produced by many different tissues, and its biological functions are diverse. Synthesized in vascular endothelium, NO dilates arteries and arterioles, regulates cardiac contractility, and inhibits platelet aggregation and adhesion (acting synergistically with prostacyclin). Evidence suggests that excess production of NO plays an important role in the pathogenesis of septic shock. NO has been identified as a neurotransmitter in the peripheral and central nervous systems and is known to relax smooth muscle. It is thought to play a role in the adaptive relaxation of the stomach, peristalsis, bronchodilatation, and also plays a part in the formation of memory. NO is generated by activated macrophages, and in high concentration has a direct cytotoxic effect. It is also an immune modulator, regulating cytokine production and inhibiting leukocyte adhesion. The NO molecules is a free radical (it has an unpaired electron) and is therefore able to scavenge superoxide ions.

1.9 (a) T (b) T (c) F (d) F (e) T

Nitric oxide synthase (NOS) exists in three isoforms, each encoded by a different gene. All forms are homodimers which oxidize the terminal guanidino group of L-arginine to form nitric oxide (NO), and also require two cosubstrates, NADPH and oxygen. NOSs have been isolated from a variety of tissues, including vascular endothelium, neurons, macrophages, neutrophils, skeletal muscle, pancreatic islet cells, endometrium, respiratory and gastrointestinal epithelium. Two of the isoforms of NOS are produced constitutively (cNOS) and are dependent on increased levels of intracellular calcium for activation. These types of NOS were originally isolated from endothelium (eNOS or NOS III) and neurons (nNOS or NOS I), although it is now known that the enzymes are distributed more widely than this. The third isoform is not produced by healthy cell types, but its production is induced by several pro-inflammatory cytokines (IL-1, IL-2, TNFα and interferon gamma). This inducible NOS (iNOS, NOS II) is synthesized by macrophages and as active at resting levels of intracellular calcium (sometimes said to be calcium-independent).

1.10 (a) F (b) T (c) T (d) T (e) F

Apolipoprotein E (apoE) is a polymorphic protein which plays an important role in the transport and metabolism of cholesterol. The apoE gene (*APOE*) is located on the long arm of chromosome 19. There are three types of apoE in humans: E2, E3 and E4. Type E3 is the most, and E2 the least, common. The alleles encoding these three types are designated ε2, ε3 and ε4. Individuals with an *APOE* ε4 allele have an increased risk of developing late-onset Alzheimer's disease with a lower age of onset. This effect is more marked in homozygotes than heterozygotes for this gene. Individuals inheriting ε2 have a reduced risk of the disease; this allele appears to be protective. ApoE is capable of binding the soluble and insoluble forms of β-amyloid protein. Both apoE and β-amyloid protein are found within senile plaques. Neurofibrillary tangles, another characteristic histopathological feature of Alzheimer's, are accumulations of abnormal neurofilaments and microtubules, a major component of which is an abnormally phosphorylated form of the microtubule protein tau.

Mutations in the gene for β-amyloid protein on chromosome 21 have been noted in some cases of familial Alzheimer's disease. Individuals over 40 years of age with Down's syndrome (trisomy 21) almost invariably have pathological evidence of Alzheimer's disease at autopsy. Other genes associated with familial Alzheimer's disease include the presenilin-1 gene (PS_1) on chromosome 14, and the presenilin-2 gene (PS_2) on chromosome 1. Families with the PS_1 gene generally have more severe disease, with earlier onset, myoclonus and language disorders. There is a positive family history of Alzheimer's disease in 20–50% of all cases, though true autosomal dominant disease accounts for only 5–10% of all cases.

1.11 (a) F (b) F (c) T (d) T (e) T

The name of this cytokine (tumour necrosis factor, TNF) is derived from experiments which showed it could induce necrosis in some tumours. It was previously named cachectin because of its association with anorexia and weight loss. The most important of the two types of TNF, TNF alpha (TNFα), is produced by macrophages. It causes fever, hypotension, hypercoagulability, upregulates leukocyte adhesion receptors on endothelial cells, enhances the microbicidal activity of macrophages and neutrophils, and regulates cell growth and apoptosis. TNFβ is synthesized by T lymphocytes, and has broadly the same actions as TNFα. The genes for TNFα and TNFβ are both located in the major histocompatibility complex class III region on chromosome 6. Increased secretion of TNF and other pro-inflammatory cytokines is responsible for the clinical syndrome of Gram-negative endotoxic shock.

1.12 (a) F (b) T (c) F (d) T (e) T

The interleukins are a group of proteins produced mainly by lymphocytes. They act mainly in a paracrine fashion, i.e. on cells in the same microenvironment. At least 15 different interleukins have been identified, acting on a variety of target tissues and having diverse functions. The major pro-inflammatory interleukins are IL-1 and IL-6 (and TNF), these being largely responsible for the features of inflammation, fever and septic shock. Some interleukins are inhibitory: IL-4, IL-10 and IL-13 promote immunoglobulin E (IgE) production, inhibit the cell-mediated immune response and suppress production of pro-inflammatory cytokines. Interleukins also function as growth and differentiation factors: IL-1 → T and B cells; IL-2 → T cells; IL3→ 'multilineage' colony stimulating factor; IL-5 → eosinophils.

1.13 (a) F (b) F (c) F (d) T (e) T

Apoptosis, or programmed cell death, is a form of cell suicide which occurs by a regulated genetic mechanism. It is important for regulating cell numbers in embryonic development, in healthy tissue, and also occurs in certain disease processes. Histologically, cells undergoing apoptosis shrink and become more dense. Chromatin becomes pyknotic and is packaged into vesicles which line the inner plasma membrane (marginalization). There is no swelling of mitochondria or other organelles. The cell membrane remains intact, but the nucleus fragments (karyorrhexis) and the cell develops numerous buds. The cell may shrink into a single dense mass (an apoptotic body) or may be phagocytosed by macrophages. The whole process is under genetic control (sometimes referred to as an internal 'clock') and is influenced by a number of proto-oncogenes, oncogenes and tumour suppressor genes, including the *p53* gene. Apoptosis can also be induced by various external agents including cytokines, hormones, natural killer (NK) cells or other toxins. In contrast, ischaemic cell death is caused by failure of the ionic pumps of the plasma membrane and is accompanied by swelling of the cell leading to necrosis and karyolysis. Ischaemic cell death induces an inflammatory response; apoptosis does not.

The commonest translocation in haematological malignancies occurs from chromosome 14 to chromosome 18 [t(14;18) (q32;q31)], creating the oncogene *bcl-2* which blocks apoptosis.

1.14 (a) F (b) F (c) T (d) F (e) T

Anti-sense oligonucleotides are short sequences of DNA which contain a complementary base sequence to a target RNA. They do not cross the plasma membrane efficiently and are delivered into the cell by cationic liposomes, microinjection or by viral vectors. The phosphodiester linkages of these oligonucleotides are modified to prevent degradation by cellular and extracellular nucleases. Within the cell, they bind (anneal) to their complementary strands of RNA, and as a result the double-stranded RNA cannot be processed, effectively blocking RNA transport, splicing or translation. This technique could be used to block transcription or translation of activated oncogenes to their oncoprotein products. Anti-sense oligonucleotides can also be used to target viral RNA (HIV, cytomegalovirus and human papilloma virus).

1.15 (a) F (b) T (c) T (d) F (e) T

Prions (proteinaceous infectious agents) are responsible for causing transmissible spongiform encephalopathies (TSEs) in a variety of animal species, including man. The agent is a glycoprotein (molecular weight 27–30 kDa) derived from a single copy gene (*prp*) on chromosome 20 which codes for a normal membrane protein (PrP^c) whose function is unclear. In prion diseases a modified form of this protein (PrP^{sc}) accumulates in neurons and neuropil, forming fibrillar amyloid plaques and vacuolation of neurons (spongiform change). PrP^{sc} is resistant to digestion by proteolytic enzymes, unlike its normal precursor PrP^c. PRP^{sc} is also resistant to degradation by heat, ionizing radiation, DNAse, RNAse, formaldehyde and disinfectants. Familial prion diseases occur as a result of mutations in the *prp* gene, but these diseases are also transmissible by a number of other routes. A number of cases of iatrogenic Creutzfeldt–Jakob disease (CJD) have been caused by administration of growth hormone (extracted from cadaveric pituitary glands), use of cadaveric dural patches in neurosurgery, and corneal grafts. It seems likely that the new variant of CJD (nvCJD) is caused by the same prion protein that causes bovine spongiform encephalopathy (BSE). Clinically, nvCJD is unlike classical CJD but bears a close resemblance in its presentation and course to kuru. Kuru is a prion disease exclusive to the Fore tribe of Papua New Guinea and is related to their practice of ritual cannibalism.

1.16 (a) F (b) T (c) F (d) T (e) F

Trinucleotide repeat diseases occur when a triplet of nucleotides (e.g. CAG) in a sequence of DNA increases in copy number. These trinucleotide repeats are usually found within, or close to, the gene associated with these diseases. When the number of triplet repeats exceeds 30–35 the DNA becomes unstable and may then expand up to several thousand copies and interfere with normal gene expression. All of these diseases exhibit anticipation – a phenomenon whereby the severity of the disease increases through successive generations and the age of onset of the disease falls. This is usually associated with an increase in the size of the repeat sequence. Genetic diseases caused by triplet repeats are shown below. Genetic imprinting refers to different expression of a gene, depending on the sex of the parent who transmits it (e.g. only the paternal copy of the insulin-like growth factor-2 (*IGF2*) gene is active in foetal development).

Trinucleotide repeat disease (triplet repeat is shown in brackets)

Autosomal dominant: Huntington's disease (CAG), myotonic dystrophy (GCT), spinocerebellar ataxia, dentatorubropallidoluyisian atrophy.
Autosomal recessive: Friedreich's ataxia.
X-linked: Fragile X syndrome (CGG), Kennedy's syndrome (X-linked bulbospinal neuropathy).

Anticipation has also been suggested in Parkinson's disease, Crohn's disease, manic depressive illness and schizophrenia.

1.17 (a) T (b) F (c) T (d) T (e) T
The p53 protein is encoded by the *p53* gene on chromosome 17 (locus 17p13.1) and is a 53 kDa nuclear phosphoprotein. It plays important roles in controlling the cell cycle, DNA synthesis and repair, cell differentiation and apoptosis. DNA damage caused by ionizing radiation stabilizes the p53 molecule and arrests the cell in the G_1 phase of the cell cycle, allowing repair of DNA strands before mitosis takes place, thus reducing the risk of mutations. Mutations in the *p53* gene are associated with most types of human cancer. Individuals with the rare, autosomal dominant Li Fraumeni syndrome inherit a single mutant copy of *p53*. As a result, they are predisposed to a spectrum of childhood and adult tumours, including carcinoma of the breast, soft tissue sarcomas, brain tumours, osteosarcomas, leukaemia, adrenocortical carcinoma and lung cancer.

1.18 (a) F (b) T (c) T (d) T (e) F
(See answer 1.19)

1.19 (a) F (b) T (c) T (d) T (e) T
The fatty acid arachidonic acid is cleaved from membrane phospholipid by the enzymes phospholipase A_2 and phospholipase C. Arachidonic acid is metabolized by two pathways: the cyclo-oxygenase pathway and the lipoxygenase pathway. The products of both pathways are termed eicosanoids. Products of the cyclo-oxygenase pathway are the prostaglandins PGD_2, PGE_2, $PGF_{2\alpha}$, PGI_2 and also thromboxane A_2 (TXA_2). The lipoxygenase pathway yields the leukotrienes LTA_4, LTB_4, LTC_4, LTD_4 and LTE_4. Glucocorticoids and some anti-malarials interfere with cleavage of arachidonic acid from the cell membrane. The enzyme cyclo-oxygenase is directly inhibited by all non-steroidal anti-inflammatory agents.

Properties of the eicosanoids

PGD_2 is a bronchoconstrictor and also plays a role in platelet aggregation and in brain function. PGE_2 is a potent inducer of bone resorption and of calcium release from bone. PGF_2 is a bronchoconstrictor and has a role in ovarian and uterine function. PGI_2 is a bronchodilator, vasodilator and inhibits platelet aggregation. TXA_2 is a bronchodilator, vasoconstrictor and enhances platelet aggregation.

Leukotrienes have histamine-like actions, including increasing vascular permeability and induction of bronchospasm. Leukotrienes are more potent bronchoconstrictors than histamine. Together LTC_4 LTD_4 and LTE_4 have been identified as the substance previously known as the slow-reacting substance of anaphylaxis (SRS-A).

1.20 (a) T (b) F (c) T (d) T (e) T

Bradykinin is a nonapeptide formed by cleavage of the plasma α-globulin molecule kininogen by the proteolytic enzyme kallikrein. Bradykinin is a potent vasodilator, activates phospholipase A to liberate arachidonic acid, and causes smooth muscle spasm in the intestine, uterus and bronchial tree. As its name suggests, its action is slower and more prolonged than histamine. Bradykinin is inactivated by the enzymes kininase I, and by angiotensin-converting enzyme in the lung.

1.21 (a) T (b) T (c) T (d) T (e) T

IL-1 was previously known as leukocyte-endogenous pyrogen, lymphocyte-activating factor, and leukocyte-endogenous mediator. IL-1 is synthesized by many cells (endothelial cells, B cells, fibroblasts), but principally by activated macrophages. IL-1 exists in two forms, α and β, which bind to α and β receptors. The receptor antagonist IL-1ra is a closely related molecule. IL-1 is one of the principal mediators of inflammation. It stimulates T cell proliferation, T cell production of IL-2, production of prostaglandins, induces production of acute phase proteins by the liver, induces fever by acting on the hypothalamus, augments corticosteroid release, and induces destructive enzymes such as collagenase. Therapeutic trials using antibodies to IL-1 and TNF have met with some success in the treatment of rheumatoid arthritis.

1.22 (a) T (b) T (c) T (d) F (e) F

Intercellular adhesion molecules are proteins which allow cell-to-cell interaction. Adhesion of leukocytes to endothelium occurs in response to tissue injury and in many immune-mediated diseases. The principal adhesion molecules are as follows.

1. The **cellular adhesion molecules (CAMs)**, which are members of the immunoglobulin superfamily and are all expressed on vascular endothelium: intracellular CAM-1 (ICAM-1), ICAM-2, vascular CAM-1 (VCAM-1) and mucosal adhesion CAM-1 (MAdCAM-1).
2. The **integrins** consist of two polypeptide chains, α and β, which are not bound covalently. β_1-Integrins are principally involved with binding leukocytes to extracellular matrix; β_2-integrins are involved in leukocyte adhesion to endothelium; β_3-integrins (cytoadhesins) have a role in the interaction of neutrophils and platelets at sites of inflammation or vascular endothelial damage.

Complement receptors 3 and 4 (CR3 and CR4) also belong to this group. CR3 and CR4 are expressed by myeloid cells and bind ICAM-1.

3. **Selectins** are transmembrane glycoproteins. This group consists of E-selectin (found on endothelial cells), P-selectin (platelets) and L-selectin (leukocytes).

Selectins and ICAMs are up-regulated by pro-inflammatory cytokines such as IL-1 and TNFα.

1.23 (a) T (b) T (c) T (d) F (e) F

Chemokines are a group of small, cysteine-rich, heparin-binding proteins released at sites of inflammation. Some of their effects are similar to cytokines, but they are distinguished by their powerful chemotactic ability. This recruitment is very specific to subgroups of leukocytes: IL-8 attracts neutrophils; RANTES attracts monocytes and memory T cells; macrophage inflammatory protein-1β (MIP-1β); MIP-1α; monocyte chemotactic peptide (MCP) and others.

Other chemotactic molecules for neutrophils include C5a, leukotriene B_4 (LTB_4) and C3a. IL-5 is a growth and differentiation factor for eosinophils.

1.24 (a) T (b) F (c) T (d) T (e) T

NK cells are lymphocytes, distinct from T and B cells. They do not express the TCR and are mostly derived from large granular lymphocytes which represent about 5% of peripheral blood leukocytes. Their function is to recognize and kill tumour cells and virus-infected cells. They can also lyse cells coated with IgG. NK cells have receptors for MHC class I molecules and the Fc fragment of IgG. NK cells secrete IFNγ, IL-1 and granulocyte macrophage-colony stimulating factor (GM-CSF).

1.25 (a) F (b) T (c) T (d) T (e) T

Mitochondria possess DNA genomes (mDNA) that are distinct from nuclear DNA. This mDNA is inherited solely from the mother: although spermatozoa are rich in mitochondria, these are confined to the tail region and do not penetrate the ovum on fertilization. Defects in mDNA give rise to a heterogenous group of disorders characterized by the presence of abnormal muscle fibrils called red ragged fibres, caused by the accumulation of abnormal mitochondria. These diseases include Kearns–Sayre syndrome, Leber's hereditary optic atrophy, Leigh disease, familial progressive external ophthalmoplegia (PEO) syndrome, MERRF syndrome (myoclonic epilepsy and red ragged fibres), MELAS syndrome (mitochondrial myopathy, encephalopathy, lactic acidosis and stroke-like episodes), succinic dehydrogenase (complex II) deficiency and cytochrome c oxidase (complex IV) deficiency.

FURTHER READING

Ackerman, M.J. and Clapham, D.E. (1997) Ion channels – basic science and clinical disease. *N Engl J Med*, **336**, 1575–85.

Alison, M.R., Wright, N.A. (1993) Growth factors and growth factor receptors. *Br J Hosp Med*, **49**, 774–90.

Askari, F.K., McDonnell, W.M. (1996) Antisense oligonucleotide therapy. *New Engl J Med* **334**, 316–19.

Bazzoni, F., Beutler, B. (1996) The tumour necrosis factor ligand and receptor families, in *Seminars in Medicine of the Beth Israel Hospital, Boston*, (ed. J.S. Flier), *New Engl J Med*, **334**, 1717–25.

Carson, D.A., Lois, A. (1995) Cancer progression and p53. *Lancet*, **346**, 1009–11.

Chen, H.L., Carbone, D.P. (1997) p53 as a target for anti-cancer immunotherapy. *Mol Med Today*, 160–7.

Clark, B., Gooi, H.C. (1994) The polymerase chain reaction (PCR) and its clinical applications. *Hospital Update*, 278–86.

Cobb, J.P. (1996) Nitric oxide and septic shock. *JAMA* **275**, 1192–6.

Cox, T.M. and Sinclair, J. (eds) (1997) *Molecular Biology in Medicine*, Blackwell Science, Oxford.

Hart, C.A. (1996) Prion diseases. *Br J Hosp Med*, **56** , 64–5.

Jackson, M. (1994) Prion diseases. *Hospital Update*, 71–80.

Krontiris, T.G. (1995) Molecular medicine: oncogenes. *New Engl J Med*, **333** 303–6.

Lefkowitz, R.J. (1995) Clinical implications of basic research: G proteins in medicine. *New Engl J Med*, **332**, 186–7.

Majno, G., Joris, I. (1995) Apoptosis, oncosis, and necrosis: an overview of cell death. *Am J Pathol*, **146**, 3–15.

Moncada, S., Higgs, A. (1993) The L-arginine–nitric oxide pathway. *New Engl J Med*, **329**, 2002–12.

Nathan, C., Xie, Q. (1994) Nitric oxide synthases: roles, tolls, and controls. *Cell* **78**, 915–18.

Post, S.G., Whitehouse, P.J., Binstock, R.H. *et al.* (1997) The clinical introduction of genetic testing for Alzheimer's disease: an ethical perspective. *JAMA*, **277** 832–6.

Savill, J. (1997) Science, medicine, and the future: molecular genetic approaches to understanding disease. *BMJ*, **314**, 126–9.

Savill, J. (1997) Science, medicine, and the future: prospecting for gold in the human genome. *BMJ* **314** 43–5.

Savill, J. (1997) Science, medicine, and the future: role of molecular biology in understanding disease. *BMJ* **314** 203–6.

Simioni, P., Prandoni, P., Lensing, A. *et al.* (1997) The risk of recurrent venous thromboembolism in patients with an $Arg^{506} \rightarrow Gln$ mutation in the gene for factor V (factor V Leiden). *New Engl J Med*, **336**, 399–403.

Tyrrell, D.A.J. (1997) Polymerase chain reaction. *BMJ*, **314** 5–6.

Wagner, R.W., Flanagan, W.M. (1997) Antisense technology and the prospects for therapy of viral infections and cancer. *Mol Med Today*, 31–8.

2 Genetics

QUESTIONS

2.1 In the thalassaemias:

(a) most patients with α^0-thalassaemia have entire deletions of α-globin genes.

(b) β^+ thalassaemia results from complete absence of β-globin chains.

(c) nonsense and frameshift mutations are usually responsible for β^0 thalassaemia.

(d) prenatal screening has reduced the incidence in areas where the disease is common.

(e) heterozygotes have an increased incidence of haematological malignancies.

2.2 The following statements regarding post-translational processing of proteins are correct:

(a) cleavage of an *N*-terminal methionine is often required to activate the protein.

(b) glycosylation takes place at the cell membrane.

(c) proteins exported from the cell are carried in Golgi vesicles to the cell membrane.

(d) conversion of proline to hydroxyproline strengthens collagen in cartilage.

(e) protein folding is dependent on chaperonins in some cases.

2.3 The following statements regarding the *BRCA-1* gene are correct:

(a) mutations are responsible for about 50% of familial breast cancers.

(b) *BRCA-1* is found on the long arm of chromosome 7.

(c) *BRCA-1* is an oncogene.

(d) mutations cause ovarian cancer only in women over 60 years.

(e) the carrier frequency of mutations is about one in 100.

2.4 In fragile X syndrome:

(a) a prenatal diagnosis can be made from a blood sample from the mother.

(b) an error rate of about 5% occurs in cytogenetic studies during prenatal screening.

(c) the condition is sometimes misdiagnosed as autism.
(d) the phenomenon of anticipation is demonstrated.
(e) mutations of the *FMR-1* gene are responsible.

2.5 Duchenne muscular dystrophy (DMD):
(a) is an autosomal recessive disorder.
(b) gene is very small.
(c) is caused by abnormal action of actin.
(d) can be diagnosed prenatally.
(e) has an incidence of about one in 3500 live births.

2.6 Mitochondrial DNA
(a) contains over 100 coding sequences.
(b) contains genes for proteins required in oxidative phosphorylation.
(c) is predominantly inherited from the father.
(d) mutation is the cause of Leber's hereditary optic neuropathy.
(e) accounts for 10% of the total human DNA.

2.7 Molecules of DNA:
(a) contain adenine, cytosine, guanine and uracil bases.
(b) are found in bacteriophages.
(c) can be detected by SDS-polyacrylamide gel electrophoresis (SDS-PAGE) and Western blotting.
(d) can be denatured at pH 4.
(e) are found in mitochondria.

2.8 Oncogenes:
(a) are expressed normally in cells during mitosis.
(b) may result from point mutation of proto-oncogenes such as *ras* genes.
(c) at the break point cluster region (bcr) of the Philadelphia chromosome are responsible for development of lymphomas.
(d) produced by insertion of viral elements are associated with the development of hepatocellular carcinoma in chronic hepatitis B infection.
(e) associated with carcinoma of the colon include *SPC* and K-*ras* molecular rearrangements.

2.9 The *p53* tumour suppressor gene:
(a) is located on the X chromosome.
(b) inhibits oncogene action in cell culture.
(c) encodes for a nuclear phosphoprotein.

(d) is mutated in many bronchial carcinomas.
(e) is a proto-oncogene.

2.10 Human gene transfer therapy:
(a) is now a standard treatment for familial hypercholesterolaemia.
(b) is only suitable for autosomal dominant disorders.
(c) for cystic fibrosis is based on modifying circulating lymphocytes to express the cystic fibrosis transmembrane regulator protein.
(d) may be achieved by human artificial chromosomes.
(e) is most efficient in highly differentiated somatic cells.

2.11 The following are inherited in an X-linked dominant manner:
(a) Turner's syndrome.
(b) Fanconi syndrome.
(c) dystrophia myotonica.
(d) vitamin D (hypophosphataemic) resistant rickets.
(e) Prader–Willi syndrome.

2.12 The following statements regarding cell division are correct:
(a) meiosis includes two cell divisions.
(b) anaphase of mitosis is identified by the coiling and condensation of DNA.
(c) after meiosis all daughter cells are genetically identical.
(d) karyotyping is best performed by arresting cell division during metaphase.
(e) triploidy (69 chromosomes) results in Patau syndrome.

2.13 If a female carrier of an X-linked recessive condition marries an asymptomatic male, the following statements are correct:
(a) half of the daughters will be symptomatic.
(b) half of the sons will be asymptomatic carriers.
(c) half of the children will be symptomatic.
(d) half of the daughters will be carriers.
(e) half of the sons will be symptomatic.

2.14 Klinefelter's syndrome is:
(a) associated with a 47 XYY karyotype.
(b) due to meiotic non-dysjunction.
(c) associated with delayed bone age.
(d) a recognized cause of hypogonadotrophic hypogonadism.
(e) inherited as an X-linked recessive disorder.

2.15 Genetic disorders which predispose to cancer include:
(a) ataxia telangiectasia.

(b) McArdle's disease.
(c) multiple endocrine neoplasia (MEN) 2a.
(d) xeroderma pigmentosa.
(e) Möbius syndrome.

2.16 A major route of metabolism for the following drugs involves genetically determined acetylation:
(a) hydralazine.
(b) sulphasalazine.
(c) nitrazepam.
(d) isoniazid.
(e) xylocaine.

2.17 DNA replication:
(a) is semi-conservative.
(b) moves in a $3' \rightarrow 5'$ direction.
(c) requires reverse transcriptase enzymes.
(d) produces an error at around one in every 1000 base pairs.
(e) occurs in a replication bubble.

2.18 Restriction fragment length polymorphisms (RFLPs):
(a) are genes for which a function has not been found.
(b) are inherited according to Mendelian genetics.
(c) can be helpful in determining the position of specific genes.
(d) are produced by enzymes which cleave DNA at specific sites.
(e) can be used in prenatal diagnosis.

2.19 The following statements concerning variations of alleles at the α_1 antitrypsin locus (α_1 protease inhibitor) are true:
(a) P_i ZZ homozygotes are likely to have emphysema.
(b) accumulation of α_1 antitrypsin in the liver is due to abnormalities of post-translational modification of the protein.
(c) P_i Z and P_i S alleles differ from P_i M by one amino acid.
(d) homozygous P_i Pittsburg variants are associated with a haemorrhage disorder.
(e) P_i ZZ phenotype is associated with an increased incidence of bronchiectasis.

2.20 Characteristic features of the genetics of bronchial asthma include:
(a) simple Mendelian recessive inheritance.
(b) an independent contribution by atopy.

(c) genetic linkage to a single chromosome.
(d) an independent contribution by bronchial hyper-responsiveness.
(e) effective study by positional cloning.

2.21 The following statements regarding cystic fibrosis are correct:
(a) in Caucasians there is a disease frequency of one in 300 live births.
(b) neonatal screening involves DNA testing for mutation analysis.
(c) there are fewer than 20 mutations of the cystic fibrosis transmembrane regulator (*CFTR*) gene described.
(d) unaffected siblings of an affected person have a two in three risk of being a carrier.
(e) the most appropriate initial test to confirm the diagnosis is the measurement of sweat sodium.

2.22 Familial hypercholesterolaemia:
(a) is an autosomal recessive disorder.
(b) homozygote individuals develop xanthomas in the first decade of life.
(c) is due to mutations of very low density lipoprotein (VLDL) receptor genes.
(d) heterozygotes have a twofold rise in cholesterol compared to unaffected individuals.
(e) heterozygotes have 15 times the increased risk of coronary artery disease compared to unaffected individuals.

2.23 Down's syndrome:
(a) has a frequency of approximately one in 700 births in the general population.
(b) has a frequency of one in 40 births at age 35 years.
(c) mosaics account for about 15% of those affected.
(d) foetuses are associated with increased blood α-fetoprotein levels in the mother.
(e) individuals have a trisomy 18 chromosomal abnormality.

2.24 Myotonic dystrophy (MD):
(a) is an autosomal recessive disorder.
(b) may present in neonates.
(c) is due to a point mutation of the MD kinase gene.
(d) increases in severity with each generation.
(e) is associated with male infertility.

2.25 Triplet repeat expansion defects account for:
(a) Huntington's disease.
(b) Friedreich's ataxia.
(c) Duchenne muscular dystrophy.
(d) fragile X syndrome.
(e) cystic fibrosis.

ANSWERS

2.1 (a) T (b) F (c) T (d) T (e) F

There has been extensive work on the genetics of the thalassaemias during the past 10–15 years. They were first described in the Mediterranean where they are common. Carriers may have an advantage in protection against the effects of malaria parasites but have no increase in the incidence of other blood disorders, including malignancies. Prenatal screening has reduced the number of live births of children with thalassaemia significantly in areas where the condition is common.

Most cases of α-thalassaemia are because of deletions of one or more genes at the α-globin gene cluster; the more deletions the greater the severity of the disease. β^0 thalassaemia, where there is complete absence of globulin, is because of nonsense and frame shift mutations. β^+ thalassaemia arises because of processing mutations.

The superscript ^{0} (e.g. α^0) thalassaemia indicates no globin production and $^+$ (e.g. α^+) indicates reduced production.

2.2 (a) T (b) F (c) T (d) T (e) T

After translation many gene products undergo further modification in the endoplasmic reticulum (ER) and Golgi apparatus. Proteolytic cleavage of *N*-terminal methionine or other signal polypeptides is a common post-translational modification. The pro-opiomelanocortin gene product may be cleaved in different ways to yield hormones such as ACTH, α-melanocyte-stimulating hormone (α-MSH), β-MSH, endorphins, lipotropin and *met*-encephalin. Proteins may be glycosylated at the ER during or after protein manufacture. Folding of proteins is important and is in some cases controlled by proteins called chaperonins. Post-translational modification of amino acid side chains such as proline to hydroxyproline in collagen is a further example of an important post-translational modification.

Proteins destined for export from the cell are released from the ER into the Golgi complex and transported to the cell membrane.

2.3 (a) T (b) F (c) F (d) F (e) F

The *BRCA-1* gene is a large gene found on chromosome 17 (long arm) and codes for an 1863-amino acid gene product which is probably a tumour suppressor gene. Over 100 mutations have been described and the carriage rate for mutations is about one in 880 (higher in Ashkenazi Jews). *BRCA-1* mutations are responsible for about 50% of breast cancers where four or more family members are affected, and also for 80% of families with a history of breast and ovarian cancer. The risk of breast and ovarian cancer is greater than 40% for individuals under 50 years who carry the *BRCA-1* gene.

2.4 (a) F (b) T (c) T (d) T (e) T

Fragile X syndrome is a common form of mental retardation affecting one in 2000 children. It derives its name from the fragile site in the X chromosome at band Xq 27.3. The clinical manifestations are quite variable and some patients with behavioural abnormalities are diagnosed as autistic. Classical dysmorphic features include facial changes and large testes. Although the condition is X-linked, about 50% of those with the fragile X site have mental retardation.

A candidate gene *FMR-1* has been isolated but its gene product is not yet identified. In families with fragile X syndrome there is increasing severity or earlier age of onset in successive generations (anticipation). This is because of the increasing size of CGG base repeats. Carriers may have five to fifty repeats, while a full mutation is over 200. This expansion leads to methylation of the gene which makes it inactive.

Prenatal screening to date has relied on cytogenetic detection in cultured amniocytes and has an overall error rate of about 5%.

2.5 (a) F (b) F (c) F (d) T (e) T

DMD has an incidence of one in 3500 live births in most populations studied. It is mostly an X-linked recessive disorder which is due to an intragenic deletion. Mutations result in failure to manufacture dystrophin which, though a minor component of muscle (<0.02% by weight), is important in anchoring the sarcolemma to actin molecules of the cytoskeleton.

Carrier screening and prenatal diagnosis is now possible for DMD. Gene transfer interventions have been tried but so far with only limited success.

2.6 (a) F (b) T (c) F (d) T (e) F

Mitochondrial DNA is small, consisting of 6569 base pairs in most populations. The DNA is tightly packed and has two ribosomal RNA genes and 22 transfer RNA genes which encode for 13 mitochondrial proteins involved in oxidative phosphorylation. Mitochondrial DNA accounts for about 0.5% of total human DNA.

Inheritance of mitochondrial DNA is primarily maternal, as sperm mitochondria are usually destroyed during fertilization. Mutations of mitochondrial DNA cause a number of rare diseases such as Leber's hereditary optic neuropathy, myoclonic epilepsy associated with ragged red fibres, Kearns–Sayre syndrome and mitochondrial encephalomyopathy, lactic acidosis and stroke-like episodes.

2.7 (a) F (b) T (c) F (d) F (e) T

DNA contains adenine, cytosine, guanine and thymidine. In RNA, thymidine is replaced by uracil. DNA is found in bacteriophages, mitochondria, chloroplasts and some viruses.

SDS-PAGE and Western blotting are used to detect protein. Northern blotting is used to detect messenger RNA using a DNA probe and Southern blotting for DNA fragments following digestion with restriction enzymes using a complimentary DNA (cDNA) probe.

DNA can be denatured at 100°C or pH $\leqslant$ 7.13. At 65°C DNA will anneal (DNA renaturation or hybridization).

2.8 (a) F (b) T (c) F (d) T (e) T

Proto-oncogenes control aspects of cellular growth and division via growth factors and their receptors, membrane and cytoplasmic transducers and DNA binding proteins (e.g. *fms* proto-oncogene forms the CSF-1 (colony stimulating factor) receptor in macrophages). Proto-oncogenes may be disrupted to produce malignant transformation by the following mechanisms:

1. Gene translocation, e.g. Philadelphia chromosome – the *c-abl* oncogene is translocated from chromosome 9 to the *bcr* region on chromosome 22. The *bcr–abl* hybrid produces a novel protein (p210) which has tyrosine kinase activity.
2. Gene amplification (e.g. *e-myc* in neuroblastoma).
3. Point mutations (e.g. K-*ras* and N-*ras* proto-oncogenes).
4. Viral insertion (e.g. hepatitis B virus and hepatocellular carcinoma).

The *SPC* and K-*ras* proto-oncogene abnormalities are associated with colonic cancer.

2.9 (a) F (b) T (c) T (d) T (e) F

The *p53* tumour suppressor gene is located on chromosome 17 and encodes for a 53 kDa protein which is a nuclear phosphoprotein and is involved in the regulation of cellular proliferation. The *p53* gene holds the cell at the G_1–S phase of the cell cycle, allowing DNA repair, and has been termed the 'cellular policeman'.

Mutations (deletion and mis-sense) of the *p53* gene are associated with carcinogenesis in the colon, lung, breast and ovary. Tumour suppressor genes are not proto-oncogenes. These are genes which promote cell division and growth.

2.10 (a) F (b) F (c) F (d) T (e) F

Human gene transfer therapy is at an early stage of development for conditions such as adenine deaminase deficiency (ADA), familial hypercholesterolaemia and cystic fibrosis. Human gene transfer therapy is most suited to:

- diseases where existing treatment options are limited;
- situations where there are suitable cells to translate (insert normal DNA). Stem cells are more efficient hosts than highly differentiated somatic cells;
- diseases caused by recessive disorders where lack of expression results in disease and a normal gene can be inserted.

Suitable vectors are viruses (e.g. retroviruses and adenovirus), plasmids, liposomes and human artificial chromosomes which may provide the safest method of gene transfer.

Gene transfer is most effective when delivered to stem cells. Differentiated cells will only express the transferred gene until their death, while stem cells will transfer the transfected gene to daughter cells.

2.11 (a) F (b) F (c) F (d) T (e) F

Turner's syndrome (45X) is usually due to monosomy X. Other structural variations may also cause this syndrome. The phenotype is short stature, webbed neck, lymphoedema and infertility.

Fanconi syndrome is due to chromosomal fragility. (It is diagnosed by increased chromosomal breakage after exposure to diepoxybutane.) The phenotype is short stature, absent radii and thumbs, pancytopenia and increased incidence of leukaemia.

Dystrophia myotonica is an autosomal dominant disorder. The phenotype includes myotonia, weakness, facial muscle atrophy, cataracts and male pattern baldness.

Hypophosphataemic rickets is an X-linked dominant disorder resulting in abnormal phosphate transport. The plasma parathyroid hormone concentrations are normal, with reduced phosphate. The phenotype includes rickets, short stature, tetany and convulsions.

Prader–Willi syndrome is a microdeletion chromosomal disorder [del (15) (911–912)]. The phenotype includes obesity, short stature and mental retardation.

2.12 (a) T (b) F (c) F (d) T (e) F
Mitosis comprises five stages:

Interphase	DNA uncoiled, chromosomes cannot be identified by light microscopy;
Prophase	coiling and condensation of DNA:
Metaphase	nuclear envelope broken down. Chromosomes moved to equatorial plate, spindle forms;
Anaphase	centromeres divide. Spindle contracts;
Telophase	nuclear envelope reforms and cytoplasm divides.

Meiosis involves two separate cell divisions. There is exchange of genetic material between homologous chromosomes during the first cell division. This is an important source of genetic variation.

Chromosomal aberrations include:

- autosomal aneuploidies, e.g. Down's syndrome, trisomy 21, Patau syndrome, trisomy 13.
- sex chromosome aneuploidies, e.g. Klinefelter's syndrome (47 XXY).
- Triploidy (69 chromosomes) and tetraploidy (92) are associated with spontaneous abortion and are incompatible with life.

2.13 (a) F (b) F (c) F (d) T (e) T
The female carrier of an X-linked recessive condition (◉) will pass the mutant chromosome on to half of her daughters who will be carriers. Half of the sons will have the condition (■) as they have a 50% chance of inheriting the mother's X chromosome. The other half will have a normal X chromosome (□) (Figure 2.1).

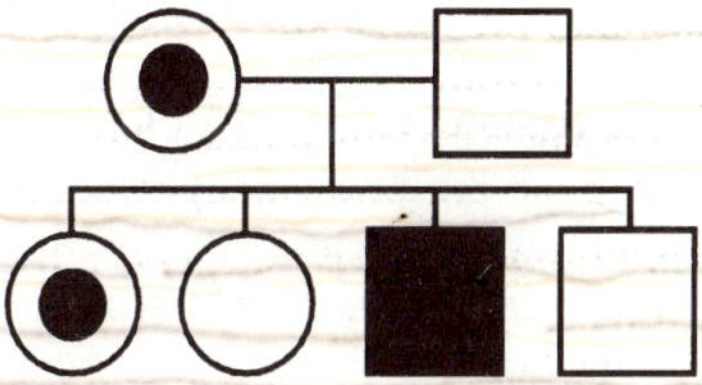

Figure 2.1 X-linked inheritance.

Mutations on the X chromosome are designated X-linked. The majority of X-linked disorders are due to recessive genes (e.g. Duchenne muscular dystrophy, haemophilia, glucose 6 phosphate dehydrogenase deficiency) and are a form of monogenic inheritance. As males carry only one X chromosome they are described as hemizygous for a particular mutant gene. During embryonic development one X chromosome is randomly suppressed in cells and so a female who is heterozygous for an abnormal gene will be a mosaic. Heterozygous females may occasionally demonstrate some features of the disease. In X-linked recessive disorders only the males are affected and females are carriers. A female carrier will transmit the disorder to half of her sons and half of her daughters will be carriers.

2.14 (a) F (b) T (c) T (d) T (e) F

The 47 XXY karyotype (Klinefelter's syndrome) is the most common cause of hypogonadism in boys. The newborn incidence is about one in 600. It is associated with mental retardation, speech and motor deficits and delayed puberty.

The 47 XYY karyotype occurs in one in 1000 male births. There is no physical phenotype. It is not associated with mental retardation though there may be hyperactivity. The cause of numerical abnormalities of chromosomes such as this is non-dysjunction during meiosis.

2.15 (a) T (b) F (c) T (d) T (e) F

Diseases associated with chromosomal fragility, e.g. Fanconi's syndrome, Bloom's syndrome, xeroderma pigmentosa and ataxia telangiectasia are associated with an increased likelihood of developing cancer. MEN 2a, an autosomal dominant disorder, is also associated with the development of tumours and is now known to be due to a mutation on chromosome 10.

2.16 (a) T (b) T (c) T (d) T (e) F

The rate at which healthy individuals metabolize drugs is genetically determined. There are a number of important pathways of metabolism which are genetically determined and which have a clinical impact.

Acetylation by the liver is determined by a recessive gene which controls the activity of *N*-acetyltransferase. Around 50% of Caucasians are slow acetylators. Slow acetylators are more likely to have adverse events to drugs metabolized by acetylation. Such patients should have a lower dose of these drugs. Examples of drugs metabolized by acetylation are dapsone, hydralazine, isoniazid, phenylzine, procainamide, nitrazepam and sulphonamides.

2.17 (a) T (b) F (c) F (d) F (e) T

DNA replication is a complex process and is semi-conservative because one strand remains conserved following separation and replication. The double helix is first unwound. The process of replication moves in a 5′ (5-prime) to 3′ (3-prime) direction and requires DNA polymerase. DNA polymerase attaches at each end of the replicating fragment and produces a replication bubble. A number of such bubbles can occur simultaneously. DNA replication is extremely accurate, with an error rate of about one in 10^9 base pairs.

2.18 (a) F (b) T (c) T (d) T (e) T

The human genome has many areas in which nucleotide sequences vary from person to person. These polymorphic areas can be used as a source of genetic markers. RFLPs are sections of DNA produced following digestion by enzymes (e.g. Taq I) which cleave DNA at variable restriction sites. RFLPs demonstrate interindividual variation and are inherited in a Mendelian fashion. They may be generated from point mutations or from GC-rich hypervariable regions.

RFLPs have been very helpful in determining where specific genes are as they are often associated with specific mutations and can be helpful in prenatal diagnosis.

2.19 (a) T (b) T (c) T (d) T (e) T

α_1 Anti-trypsin (also called α_1 protease inhibitor (α_1PI)) is an important serine protease inhibitor and part of the serpin superfamily of proteins. The protein is a product of a highly polymorphic locus with over 75 alleles recognized. The common or wild type is P_i M.

P_i Z and P_i S variants are associated with lung (emphysema and bronchiectasis) and liver disease. The lung disease (mostly emphysema) is due to proteolysis of elastin and other matrix proteins by uninhibited elastase. Liver disease is due to the accumulation of abnormally folded protein in hepatocytes. This is due to a post-translation defect at the level of the rough endoplasmic reticulum, resulting in abnormal tertiary conformation. A rare variant P_i Pittsburg, due to substitution of a methionine by an arginine residue, inhibits thrombin and results in a severe haemorrhagic disorder.

2.20 (a) F (b) T (c) F (d) T (e) F

Asthma is inherited as a complex trait. Total immunoglobulin E (IgE) (atopy) and bronchial hyper-responsiveness are quantifiable and closely associated traits associated with the clinical expression of asthma. Methods used to identify the mode of inheritance and genetic loci for asthma include segregation and linkage analyses.

Candidate genes for hyper-responsiveness and total IgE have been localized to 5q31–33. This region includes various interleukins, the β_2 adrenergic receptor and GM-CSF and G-CSF. Fine mapping will be required to locate the precise position of these genes.

2.21 (a) F (b) F (c) F (d) T (e) T

Cystic fibrosis is the most common fatal autosomal recessive disorder in North West European populations. The carrier rate for mutations of the cystic fibrosis transmembrane regulator (*CFTR*) gene is about one in 25 of the population. The disease frequency is about one in 2500 live births. Prenatal screening employed linkage disequilibrium analysis prior to the description of the *CFTR* gene, but now gene analysis for common mutations is used. There are over 400 mutations at the *CFTR* locus described (chromosome 7) and most laboratories screen for about nine. Neonatal screening relies on the measurement of immunoreactive trypsin (IRT) from a heel stab blood sample. A positive IRT test needs to be repeated and a diagnosis of cystic fibrosis cannot be made without a diagnostic sweat test.

The risk of inheritance of cystic fibrosis, if both parents are carriers, is one in four, and the risk of a child being a carrier is two in four.

2.22 (a) F (b) T (c) F (d) T (e) F

Familial hypercholesterolaemia is an autosomal dominant trait. Mutations of the low density lipoprotein (LDL) receptor result in an inability to take LDLs, a major cholesterol carrier, from the liver into the peripheral tissues.

Failure of receptor-mediated endocytosis results in an approximately twofold increase in serum cholesterol, and a four to fivefold increase in the incidence of coronary artery disease. Homozygotes have virtually no LDL receptor activity and develop xanthomas early in life, and heart disease in the second or third decade.

2.23 (a) T (b) F (c) F (d) F (e) F

Down's syndrome or trisomy 21 (47XX, +21 for a female) is due to a chromosomal non-disjunction during meiosis. A non-disjunction during mitosis in the developing embryo results in mosaicism and this accounts for about 2% of Down's syndrome individuals. The incidence of trisomy 21 in the population is about one in 700 live births. Most births occur in younger women but the rate increases steeply after the age of 35 years and is about one in 40 after 40 years of age.

Screening in pregnancy now involves the 'triple test' of alpha-fetoprotein (decreased), oestriol (decreased) and human chorionic gonadotrophin (increased); low values for all three suggest trisomy 18, Edward's syndrome. This test will detect 60% of cases of Down's syndrome, with a high false-positive rate, and amniocentesis is required to confirm the diagnosis. Tests based on foetal cell analysis from the maternal circulation may prove more accurate than hormonal tests.

2.24 (a) F (b) T (c) F (d) T (e) T
Myotonic dystrophy (MD) is due to a GCT repeat expansion at the 3′ untranslated region of the MD kinase gene on chromosome 19. The length of the repeat usually increases in each generation and is related to increased severity (anticipation). Males are infertile. Severe infantile MD occurs with maternal transmission of the gene and about 20% of children of an affected mother manifest this form of the disease. It is an autosomal dominant disorder.

Clinical features include myotonia, muscular weakness, cataracts, diabetes mellitus, cardiac arrhythmias, gonadal atrophy and infertility, early menopause and frontal balding.

2.25 (a) T (b) T (c) F (d) T (e) F
The following are examples of diseases caused by expansion of an unstable triplet of repeat sequences in a gene causing disease: Huntington's disease (CAG repeats), fragile X-syndrome, myotonic dystrophy, spinal and bulbar muscle atrophy, spinocerebellar ataxia, Friedreich's ataxia and Machado–Joseph disease.

The base triplet increases with each generation, as does the severity of the disease (anticipation).

FURTHER READING

Connor, M. and Ferguson-Smith, M. (1997) *Essential Medical Genetics*, Blackwell Scientific Publications, London.

Healy, B. (1997) *BrcA* genes – bookmaking, fortune-telling and medical care. *N Eng J Med*, **336** 1448.

Weatherall, D.J. (1991) *The New Genetics and Clinical Practice*, Oxford University Press, Oxford.

3 Clinical chemistry

QUESTIONS

3.1 The oxygen affinity of haemoglobin is:

(a) increased by a rise in the level of 2,3 diphosphoglycerate (DPG).
(b) reduced by a fall in temperature.
(c) increased by a fall in pH.
(d) independent of the $P\text{O}_2$.
(e) greater for HbA than for foetal haemoglobin (HbF).

3.2 The following statements regarding the metabolism of iron are correct:

(a) the average adult daily requirement is approximately 2 mg/day.
(b) the daily iron loss in an adult male is approximately 1 mg/day.
(c) iron is principally absorbed in the terminal ileum.
(d) iron absorption is increased in aplastic anaemia.
(e) absorption is facilitated by tetracycline.

3.3 Regarding iron storage:

(a) in an adolescent, tissue stores contain more iron than the circulating haemoglobin.
(b) serum ferritin concentration correlates well with iron stores.
(c) ferritin synthesis is stimulated by iron.
(d) haemosiderin is mobilized from iron stores in preference to ferritin.
(e) both ferritin and haemosiderin stain blue with potassium ferricyanide (Prussian blue).

3.4 Transferrin:

(a) carries iron in the ferric (Fe^{3+}) form.
(b) is normally 80% saturated with iron.
(c) levels are raised in pregnancy.
(d) levels are raised in haemochromatosis.
(e) may be saturated in aplastic anaemia.

3.5 Total iron-binding capacity (TIBC) may be increased in:

(a) iron deficiency anaemia.
(b) chronic infection.
(c) sideroblastic anaemia.

(d) women taking the oral contraceptive pill.
(e) viral hepatitis.

3.6 In a patient with acute renal impairment, the following results would suggest a pre-renal rather than a renal cause:
(a) urine osmolality > 550 mosm/kg.
(b) urine urea < 150 mmol/24h.
(c) urine sodium < 20 mmol/l.
(d) hyperkalaemia.
(e) presence of red cell casts in the urine on light microscopy.

3.7 Causes of high plasma urea: creatinine ratio include:
(a) dehydration.
(b) rhabdomyolysis.
(c) steroids.
(d) cimetidine.
(e) gastrointestinal haemorrhage.

3.8 Elevated levels of thyroxine-binding globulin (TBG) may be associated with:
(a) acromegaly.
(b) pregnancy.
(c) nephrotic syndrome.
(d) chronic liver disease.
(e) treatment with high-dose steroids.

3.9 The following findings would support a diagnosis of benign paraproteinaemia:
(a) paraprotein concentration of 50 g/l.
(b) fewer than five lytic lesions on a skull radiograph.
(c) no Bence–Jones proteins in the urine.
(d) immunoglobulin A (IgA) paraproteinaemia.
(e) plasma calcium of 3.2 mmol/l.

3.10 Bence–Jones proteins:
(a) typically consist of immunoglobulin heavy chains.
(b) are invariably associated with a serum paraproteinaemia.
(c) may be associated with a benign monoclonal gammopathy.
(d) can be reliably tested for using urine dipsticks.
(e) may cause renal amyloidosis.

3.11 Regarding magnesium metabolism:
(a) magnesium is mainly located in the extracellular space.
(b) magnesium is primarily absorbed in the ileum and jejunum.

(c) fresh fruit is a rich source of magnesium.
(d) parathyroid hormone (PTH) directly increases renal tubular reabsorption of magnesium.
(e) thiazides cause greater renal excretion of magnesium than loop diuretics.

3.12 Causes of hypomagnesaemia include:
(a) primary aldosteronism.
(b) hypoparathyroidism.
(c) cisplatin.
(d) end-stage renal failure.
(e) villous adenoma of the colon.

3.13 Alpha-1-antitrypsin (α_1-AT):
(a) is an acute phase protein.
(b) is synthesized by the liver.
(c) activity is greatly increased by cigarette smoke.
(d) levels in ZZ homozygotes are typically 80% of normal.
(e) deficiency is associated with an increased risk of emphysema.

3.14 The following findings may be considered normal in a pregnant woman at 36 weeks' gestation:
(a) low mean red cell volume (MCV).
(b) raised serum thyroid hormone-binding globulin (TBG) concentration.
(c) plasma sodium concentration of 130 mmol/l.
(d) folmerular filtration rate of 150 ml/min.
(e) glycosuria.

3.15 Methaemoglobinaemia may be caused by:
(a) nitroglycerine.
(b) primaquine.
(c) potassium chlorate.
(d) amyl nitrite.
(e) methylene blue.

3.16 According to the Friedrickson/WHO classification of hyperlipidaemia:
(a) type I may be due to a deficiency of apoprotein C.
(b) plasma very low density lipoprotein (VLDL) levels are elevated in type IV.
(c) inheritance of type IIb is autosomal recessive.
(d) type III is associated with an increased risk of developing ischaemic heart disease.
(e) pancreatitis is a recognized complication of type IIa.

3.17 Parathyroid hormone-related peptide (PTHrP):
(a) shares a common receptor with parathormone (PTH).
(b) is indistinguishable from PTH on radioimmunoassay.
(c) decreases renal tubular reabsorption of calcium.
(d) is produced in large quantities within sarcoid granulomata.
(e) levels in the plasma may be increased in carcinoma of the bronchus.

3.18 In a patient with congenital adrenal hyperplasia (CAH) because of 21-hydroxylase deficiency, plasma levels of the following substances will be elevated:
(a) sodium.
(b) adrenocorticotrophic hormone (ACTH).
(c) 17α-hydroxyprogesterone.
(d) 11-deoxycortisol.
(e) aldosterone.

3.19 The following statements regarding autoantibodies in connective tissue diseases are true:
(a) anti-Jo_1 antibodies are associated with polymyositis.
(b) anti-centromere antibodies are strongly associated with limited cutaneous scleroderma (CREST).
(c) anti-U_1RNP antibodies are typically associated with mixed connective tissue disease.
(d) presence of anti-Sm antibody is highly specific for systemic lupus erythematosus.
(e) transplacental transfer of anti-Ro antibodies commonly results in neonatal congenital heart block.

3.20 The following biochemical findings are typical of acromegaly:
(a) failure of growth hormone (GH) levels to suppress after an oral glucose tolerance test.
(b) failure of GH levels to rise in response to insulin-induced hypoglycaemia.
(c) a fall in the serum GH level in response to an intravenous infusion of arginine.
(d) raised serum levels of insulin-like growth factor 1 (IGF-1).
(e) hypercalciuria.

3.21 Urinary levels of the following substances will be elevated in an acute episode of acute intermittent porphyria:
(a) porphobilinogen (PBG).
(b) uroporphyrinogen.
(c) protoporphyrinogen.

(d) aminolaevulinic acid (ALA).
(e) coproporphyrinogen.

3.22 The presence in the plasma of anti-neutrophil cytoplasmic antibodies (ANCA) may be associated with:
(a) giant cell arteritis.
(b) Churg–Strauss syndrome.
(c) Kawasaki disease.
(d) microscopic polyarteritis.
(e) primary sclerosing cholangitis.

3.23 The following statements regarding calcium and phosphate homeostasis are true:
(a) the action of ultraviolet light on the skin catalyses the 1α-hydroxylation of 25-hydroxycholecalciferol.
(b) parathormone (PTH) increases renal reabsorption of calcium.
(c) PTH is phosphaturic.
(d) calcitonin inhibits osteoclast-mediated bone resorption.
(e) hypocalcaemia is a frequent complication of medullary carcinoma of the thyroid gland.

3.24 Characteristic early features of acute salicylate poisoning include:
(a) respiratory alkalosis.
(b) hyperkalaemia.
(c) lactic acidosis.
(d) passage of urine with $pH > 6$.
(e) tinnitus.

3.25 The Haemoccult card (guaiac) used for testing faecal occult blood:
(a) utilizes the peroxidase-like activity of haemoglobin.
(b) is able to detect gastrointestinal blood loss of 2–3 ml per day.
(c) may give a false–positive result in patients taking ferrous sulphate.
(d) may give a false–positive result in patients taking vitamin C.
(e) is more sensitive for left-sided than right-sided colonic tumours.

ANSWERS

3.1 (a) F (b) F (c) F (d) F (e) F
A shift of the haemoglobin dissociation curve to the right causes a reduction in the affinity of haemoglobin for oxygen. Physiological

mechanisms which decrease oxygen affinity, allowing increased oxygen delivery to tissues, include rises in the H^+ concentration (fall in pH), the P_{CO_2} (the Bohr effect), red cell 2,3-DPG concentration and temperature.

Haemoglobins with high oxygen affinities have their dissociation curves shifted to the left. As a result there is less oxygen released to the tissues at low partial pressures. HbF has a higher affinity for oxygen than HbA, thereby allowing transplacental transfer of oxygen from mother to foetus. Other haemoglobins which have a higher oxygen affinity than HbA include methaemoglobin and carboxyhaemoglobin. Haemoglobin S has a lower oxygen affinity than HbA.

3.2 (a) T (b) T (c) F (d) F (e) F

The average daily iron intake of an adult is 14 mg/day, of which only about 10% is usually absorbed. Liver, meat and cereals are rich sources of iron. Free iron in the gut (in the Fe^{2+} form) is absorbed into mucosal cells of the proximal small intestine. Absorption is increased by gastric acid, vitamin C (ascorbic acid), alcohol and by increased haemopoiesis. Absorption may increase to 30% of the total iron intake in severe iron deficiency. Absorption is decreased by tetracycline, achlorhydria, tannin, phytates and phosphates. Within the cells of the intestinal mucosa iron is oxidized to the Fe^{3+} form before being combined with apoferritin to form ferritin – the main form in which iron is stored in the bone marrow, liver and spleen. Iron is carried in the blood bound to transferrin.

The total body iron content is approximately 4 g, 70% of which is in the form of haem. The average iron loss is 1 mg/day, principally through the gastrointestinal tract as the intestinal mucosa desquamates. Some loss occurs through the skin. There is an additional average daily loss of 1 mg/day in menstruating women. The loss during pregnancy is approximately 1.5 mg/day. There is a diurnal variation in the serum iron, with the highest levels in the morning and the lowest in the evening.

3.3 (a) F (b) T (c) T (d) F (e) T

Ferritin, the main storage form of iron, is a water-soluble protein–iron complex (molecular weight 465 000) synthesized by the liver. Synthesis is stimulated by iron. Ferritin is composed of 24 polypeptide sub-units which form an outer protein shell (apoferritin) surrounding an inner core of ferric phosphate and hydroxide. Each apoferritin molecule is able to bind approximately 4000 atoms of iron. Iron atoms enter or leave the complex via six channels in the protein shell and are therefore readily available for use. Haemosiderin is derived from ferritin but has a higher iron content, forming insoluble deposits in the cytoplasm. The iron from haemosiderin is not easily mobilized. Deposits of both ferritin and haemosiderin are visible on light microscopy after staining with potassium ferricyanide (Prussian blue or Perl's stain).

There is a close correlation between serum ferritin concentration and body iron stores, with 1 µg/l serum ferritin equivalent to about 10 mg stored iron. Ferritin levels are high in neonates, iron overload, cancer, liver disease, infection and inflammation (ferritin is an acute phase protein). Depleted iron stores are common during the growth spurts of infancy and adolescence, and in pregnancy.

3.4 (a) T (b) F (c) T (d) F (e) T

Before incorporation into transferrin, any free iron in the plasma must be oxidized from the Fe^{2+} (ferrous) to the Fe^{3+} (ferric) form by caeruloplasmin. Transferrin (molecular weight 80 000) is a single-chain polypeptide with two binding sites for Fe^{3+}. Transferrin is usually about one-third saturated with iron, and transferrin saturation therefore regulates iron absorption. When iron stores become depleted the transferrin saturation in the blood falls. Transferrin interacts with specific receptors on the surface of erythroblasts and reticulocytes, transferring iron atoms to a carrier protein. The iron atoms are incorporated into molecules of protoporphyrin IX by the enzyme ferrochelatase, to form haem. Mature erythrocytes are incapable of further iron uptake since the transferrin-specific cell surface receptors are lost when haemoglobin synthesis is complete.

Increased transferrin saturation occurs in iron overload (e.g. multiply transfused patients, haemochromatosis), in haemolysis, severe liver disease and in bone marrow hypo- or aplasia (because of reduced iron utilization). Transferrin levels in these conditions are typically normal or reduced. Transferrin levels are increased in iron deficiency, in pregnancy and by the oral contraceptive pill.

3.5 (a) T (b) F (c) F (d) T (e) T

Transferrin binds most of the serum iron and thus the TIBC is directly related to serum transferrin levels. Iron deficiency anaemia is characterized by low serum iron levels and a high or normal TIBC. In anaemia of chronic disease (chronic infection, inflammation or malignancy), the serum iron may be low, but the TIBC is reduced. Since transferrin levels are increased in pregnancy and by the oral contraceptive pill, the TIBC is also increased. In thalassaemia the TIBC is low because of haemolysis, ineffective erythropoiesis and repeated transfusions (Table 3.1).

Table 3.1 Abnormalities of iron storage and transport

Disorder	Serum iron	Transferrin	TIBC	Ferritin
Iron deficiency anaemia	↓	↑	↑	↓
Chronic disease	↓	↓/Normal	↓/Normal	↑
Pregnancy	↓	↑	↑	↓
Oral contraceptive pill	Normal	↑	↑	Normal
Sideroblastic anaemia	↑	Normal	Normal	↑
Thalassaemia	↑/Normal	↓	↓	↑/Normal
Acute viral hepatitis	Normal	↑	↑	↑
Haemochromatosis	↑	↓	↓	↑

3.6 (a) T (b) F (c) T (d) F (e) F

Pre-renal failure is usually caused by circulatory collapse (e.g. hypovolaemia, cardiac failure, haemorrhage, hypotension or severe burns). Renal hypoperfusion reduces the glomerular filtration rate (GFR) and thereby stimulates the renin–angiotensin–aldosterone system, producing a small volume of concentrated urine with a low sodium concentration (Table 3.2). Although tubular function is normal, urea and creatinine are retained because of the low GFR. Acidosis and hyperkalaemia are the result of diminished delivery of sodium to the distal tubule, but are also features of intrinsic renal failure (acute tubular necrosis). If untreated, pre-renal failure may progress to acute tubular necrosis.

Table 3.2 Pre-renal failure

	Pre-renal failure	**Renal failure**
Urine volume	Low	Low
Urine sodium	< 20 mmol/l	> 40 mmol/l
Urine area	> 350 mmol/24 h	< 150 mmol/24 h
Urine osmolality	> 550 mosm/kg	< 350 mosm/kg
Urine : plasma urea	> 10 : 1	< 3 : 1
Urine : plasma osmolality	> 1.5 : 1	< 1.1 : 1
Urea : creatinine	> 20 : 1	< 15 : 1

3.7 (a) T (b) F (c) T (d) F (e) T

↑Urea: creatinine ratio	**↑Creatinine: urea ratio**
Dehydration	Liver failure
Gastrointestinal haemorrhage	Pregnancy
Steroids	Haemodialysis
Tetracycline	Rhabdomyolysis
Muscle wasting	Increased muscle bulk
High protein intake	Trimethoprim
	Cimetidine
	Low protein intake

3.8 (a) F (b) T (c) F (d) F (e) F

Conditions associated with altered concentration of TBG follow:

Raised TBG	**Low TBG**
Hypothyroidism	Hyperthyroidism
Pregnancy	Testosterone/androgens
Acute hepatitis	Glucocorticoid excess
Acute intermittent porphyria	Chronic liver disease
Oestrogens and oral contraceptive pill	Acromegaly
Tamoxifen	Nephrotic syndrome
Clofibrate	
Heroin/methadone	

3.9 (a) F (b) F (c) T (d) F (e) F

A paraprotein is an immunoglobulin secreted by a single clone of B lymphocytes or plasma cells. The paraprotein separates into a band, usually in the γ-region, on serum electrophoresis. Multiple myeloma is most frequently associated with paraproteins of IgG (55%) or IgM (22%) type. Waldenström's macroglobulinaemia is characterized by an IgM paraprotein. Paraproteins may also occur in B cell lymphoma and in chronic lymphocytic leukaemia.

Benign paraproteinaemia occurs in approximately 1% of the population aged over 50 years, and in 10% aged over 70 years. Patients with benign monoclonal gammopathies usually have a paraprotein concentration of < 20 g/l, no Bence–Jones proteins in the urine, no suppression of normal immunglobulin levels, no lytic bone lesions, less than 5% bone marrow plasmocytosis, and no anaemia, renal failure or hypercalcaemia. The paraprotein should remain at a constant level when the patient is followed up over a period of years. Myeloma may develop in 11% of patients with benign monoclonal gammopathy.

3.10 (a) F (b) F (c) F (d) F (e) T

Bence–Jones proteins are dimers of immunoglobulin light chains of either kappa (κ) or lambda (λ) and are present in the urine of about 50% of all cases of myeloma. Patients secreting lambda light chains have a significantly shorter survival than those secreting kappa light chains, possibly because lambda chains are more likely to cause renal damage and amyloid than kappa chains. Light chain disease, in which only light chains are produced by the plasma cell clones, occurs in 20% of cases of myeloma, and is not associated with a serum paraprotein. Myeloma heavy chain disease is rare and not associated with Bence–Jones proteinuria or nephrotoxicity.

Dipsticks for testing urine are not reliable for testing for the presence of light chains. Bence–Jones proteins are best detected by electrophoresis of a concentrated urine specimen.

3.11 (a) F (b) T (c) F (d) T (e) F

Magnesium is an intracellular cation, with 50% of the body's stores located in bone. Most is bound to adenosine triphosphate (ATP) within the cell, and this magnesium–ATP complex acts as an essential co-factor for numerous enzyme systems. The daily magnesium requirement is 10 mmol (250 mg); rich sources include seed grain, nuts, peas and beans. Fresh meat, fish and fruit have a low magnesium content. Of the magnesium ingested, 30–40% is absorbed in the ileum and jejunum. Renal conservation of magnesium is controlled by both PTH (directly) and aldosterone: 25% is reabsorbed in the proximal tubule and 50–60% in the loop of Henlé. Loop diuretics will therefore cause greater renal excretion of magnesium than thiazides acting on the distal tubule.

Hypomagnesaemia seldom occurs in isolation and is frequently associated with hypocalcaemia and hypokalaemia. Mild hypomagnesaemia may be associated with increased PTH secretion, but very low plasma magnesium levels (< 0.4 mmol/l) block release of PTH and also induce end-organ resistance to this hormone. In such cases hypocalcaemia only responds to magnesium replacement. Magnesium levels should always be measured in hypocalcaemic patients who fail to respond to treatment. The mechanism for hypokalaemia in hypomagnesaemic patients is less well understood.

3.12 (a) T (b) T (c) T (d) F (e) T

The clinical features of hypomagnesaemia include muscle weakness, tetany, convulsions, confusion, ataxia, chorea and arrhythmias. Arrhythmias are commoner when hypomagnesaemia and hypokalaemia occur together, and may include ventricular tachycardia, torsade des pointes and ventricular fibrillation. Causes of hypomagnesaemia include:

Nutrition	Malnutrition, total parenteral nutrition (without supplementation)
Gastrointestinal	Malabsorption, chronic diarrhoea, steatorrhoea
Endocrine	Hypo- and hyperparathyroidism, primary aldosteronism, diabetic ketoacidosis
↑ Renal excretion	Drugs: cisplatin, aminoglycoside antibiotics, amphotericin B, diuretics (loop and thiazides), pentamidine, theophylline toxicity, ethanol ingestion, recovery phase of acute tubular necrosis
Chronic alcoholism	

Hypermagnesaemia is associated with severe chronic renal failure.

3.13 (a) T (b) T (c) F (d) F (e) T

Alpha-1-antitrypsin (α_1-AT) is a naturally occurring protease inhibitor, encoded on chromosome 14 and synthesized by the liver. Homozygotes for the normal enzyme are designated Pi MM (Pi, protease inhibitor). The most common mutant alleles are the S and Z types – both are due to single amino acid substitutions.

Levels of α_1-AT are less than 10% of normal in ZZ and SS homozygotes. These individuals develop severe panacinar emphysema in the third and fourth decades of life. MZ and SZ heterozygotes also show some susceptibility. Emphysema has a much earlier onset in smokers: cigarette smoke oxidizes the active site of the α_1-AT molecule such that what little normal enzyme is present is less effective. Since α_1-AT normally constitutes 90% of the α_1-globulin band on serum electrophoresis, α_1-AT deficiency is strongly suggested by the absence of this band.

The abnormal proteins accumulate in the hepatocyte, causing liver damage and ultimately cirrhosis. Liver disease is also more common in ZZ and SS homozygotes.

3.14 (a) F (b) T (c) T (d) T (e) T

Haematological changes

During pregnancy the plasma volume increases progressively, peaking during the third trimester at 45% above non-pregnant values. Meanwhile, the total red cell mass increases by 25% – the net effect being haemodilution, resulting in low haemoglobin, packed cell volume and red cell count. The mean cell haemoglobin concentration remains at non-pregnant values and there is a slight increase in the MCV. A fall in the MCV is often the first indication of iron deficiency. Transferring levels are double their normal value, and therefore total iron-binding capacity (TIBG) is increased. Ferritin levels steadily decline through pregnancy.

Biochemical changes

Glomerular filtration rate (GFR) increases by 50% (normal value around 120 ml/min in non-pregnant women). Plasma urea and creatinine typically fall from normal values by 1.2 mmol/l and 22 μmol/l, respectively. Since total body water increases by 6–8 l the plasma osmolality is reduced and plasma sodium falls by 3–6 mmol/l from normal. Plasma potassium stays within the normal range. Glycosuria occurs because of the increased filtered load of glucose and decreased absorption by the proximal convoluted tubule. Lactosuria may also occur. Lipid biochemistry is altered: there is increased triglyceride (very low density lipoprotein (VLDL)) and high density lipoprotein (HDL) cholesterol, while plasma low density lipoprotein (LDL) is reduced. Serum alkaline phosphatase is elevated because of production of the placental isoenzyme. Serum TBG is double that of non-pregnant values. Free thyroxine (fT4) and tri-iodothyronine (fT3) remain normal, though total T3 and T4 are elevated.

3.15 (a) T (b) T (c) T (d) T (e) F

Methaemoglobin contains iron which has been oxidized to the ferric (Fe^{3+}) state. The degree of cyanosis produced by 1.5 g/dl of methaemoglobin is equivalent to that produced by 5 g/dl of deoxygenated haemoglobin. Levels of methaemoglobin above 10–20% of the total haemoglobin are usually associated with symptoms of dyspnoea or headache. Methaemoglobinaemia is treated with methylene blue. Methaemoglobinaemia has genetic and acquired causes.

Genetic causes are cytochrome b_5 reductase deficiency (autosomal recessive) and abnormal haemoglobin variants; all are designated HbM, e.g. HbM Boston or HbM Milwaukee (all autosomal dominant). They are due to abnormalities in either the α or β chain.

Acquired causes are chemicals and drugs which oxidize ferrous iron. Chemicals include nitrites and nitrates (sodium nitrite, amyl nitrite, nitroglycerin, nitroprusside and silver nitrate), chlorates, chromate, ferricyanide, quinones and aniline dyes. Drugs include phenacetin, primaquine, sulphonamides and dapsone.

3.16 (a) T (b) T (c) F (d) F (e) F

Type I hyperlipidaemia is due to hyperchylomicronaemia (triglyceride). The underlying defect is deficiency of lipoprotein lipase or apoprotein C. It is inherited as autosomal recessive. Usually presenting in childhood, clinical features may include acute pancreatitis, lipaemia retinalis, eruptive xanthomata and hepatosplenomegaly. There is no increased risk of ischaemic heart disease (IHD).

Type IIa (familial hypercholesterolaemia) is inherited as autosomal dominant and is because of a defect in the low density lipoprotein (LDL) receptor. This results in high LDL (cholesterol) levels. Clinical features include tendon xanthomata, xanthelasma, corneal arcus senilis and a large joint polyarthropathy. There is a strong association with IHD; untreated homozygotes have a life expectancy of 30 years. Homozygotes are also predisposed to supravalvular aortic stenosis because of formation of massive xanthomata in the ascending aorta.

Type IIb (mixed hyperlipidaemia) is associated with raised LDL and VLDL (cholesterol and triglyceride). It has an autosomal dominant inheritance. Clinical features include xanthelasma and corneal arcus senilis. There is an increased risk of IHD.

Type III (remnant disease) is due to an abnormality of apoprotein E. As a result plasma levels of intermediate density lipoprotein (IDL) (cholesterol and triglyceride) are increased. Palmar xanthomata and tuberous xanthomata are unique to type III. Other clinical features include xanthelasmas, diabetes mellitus, gout, hepatosplenomegaly and an increased risk of generalized atherosclerosis.

Type IV (familial hypertriglyceridaemia) is associated with raised plasma VLDL (triglyceride). It has an autosomal dominant inheritance. Classically patients have a triad of obesity, hyperglycaemia and hyperinsulinaemia. Clinical features include eruptive xanthomata, acute pancreatitis, lipaema retinalis, gout, hepatosplenomegaly, peripheral neuropathy and dementia. There is an increased risk of atheromatous disease.

Type IV hyperlipidaemia is a combination of types I and IV (chylomicrons and VLDL).

3.17 (a) T (b) F (c) F (d) F (e) T

PTHrP is a 141-amino acid hormone (molecular weight 16 000) with its gene located on the short arm of chromosome 12. The PTH gene is on chromosome 11. It shares close sequence homology with PTH at the amino terminal end of the molecule: both PTH and PTHrP act on PTH receptors to decrease renal excretion of calcium and to increase bone resorption. Tumours which secrete PTHrP include squamous cell carcinomas (lung and oesophagus), renal, breast, ovary, pancreas, skin and bladder carcinomas and lymphomas. It is said to cause humoral hypercalcaemia since it may cause hypercalcaemia in the absence of skeletal metastases. Biochemical effects include hypercalcaemia, hypophosphataemia and increased urinary cyclic AMP. Modern two-site radioimmunoassays (which detect whole molecules) can readily differentiate between PTH and PTHrP. PTHrP is also thought to be important in maintaining a calcium gradient across the placenta.

The hypercalcaemia of sarcoidosis is because of production of the active metabolite of vitamin D (1,25-dihydroxycholecalciferol) within granulomata.

3.18 (a) F (b) T (c) T (d) F (e) F

Deficiency of 21-hydroxylase is the most common form of CAH, accounting for 95% of cases in the UK (Figure 3.1). The disease is frequently incomplete such that increased ACTH secretion maintains adequate cortisol levels. Cases of complete deficiency present in early childhood with salt loss and virilization. Females have ambiguous genitalia. The diagnosis is made by confirming increased plasma levels of the enzyme substrate, 17α-hydroxyprogesterone (Table 3.3).

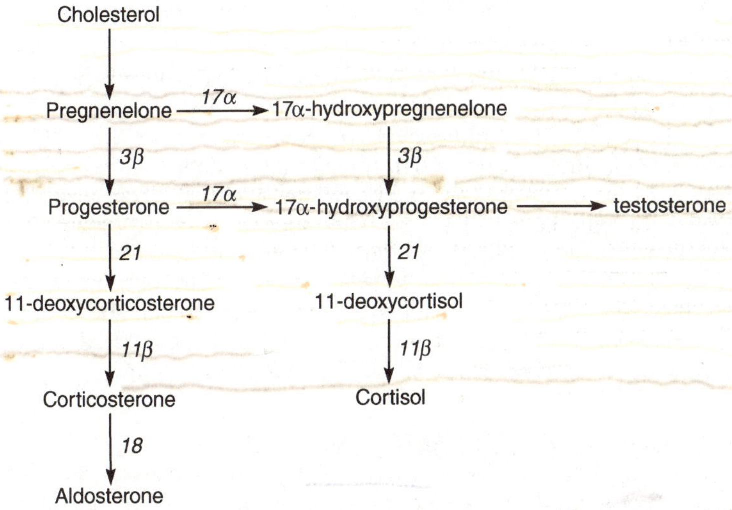

Figure 3.1 Pathways of aldosterone, cortisol and testosterone synthesis.

11β-hydroxylase deficiency accounts for most of the remaining 5% of cases of CAH. 17α-hydroxylase and 3β-hydroxydehydrogenase deficiency are rare.

Table 3.3 Symptoms of congenital adrenal hyperplasia

	3β	21-OH	11β-OH	17α-OH
Salt loss	+	+	–	–
Virilization	–	+	+	–
Hypertension	–	–	+	+
Ambiguous genitalia				
Male	+	–	–	+
Female	+	+	+	–

3.19 (a) T (b) T (c) T (d) T (e) F

Antibody	**Disease**
Anti-dsDNA	Systemic lupus erythematosus (SLE)
Anti-Sm	SLE
Anti-U_1RNP	Mixed connective tissue disease
Anti-Ro (SSA)	SLE, Sjögren's
Anti-La (SSB)	SLE, Sjögren's
Anti-centromere	Limited scleroderma (CREST)
Anti-Scl-70	Systemic sclerosis
Anti-Jo_1	Polymyositis

A number of autoantibodies and extractable nuclear antigens are associated with SLE. Anti-nuclear antibodies (ANA) are seen in 95% of patients with SLE. Anti-dsDNA is fairly specific for SLE and is seen in some 70% of cases. High titres of anti-dsDNA antibodies are associated with disease activity and with nephritis. Transplacental transfer of maternal anti-Ro antibodies may result in a transient skin rash in the neonate, but congenital heart block is rare. Patients with subacute cutaneous lupus may be ANA-negative, but most have anti-Ro or ssDNA antibodies and are HLA DR3. Renal and central nervous system involvement is not typical. In drug-induced lupus, patients all have ANA, but anti-dsDNA antibodies are rare.

3.20 (a) T (b) F (c) F (d) T (e) T

Acromegaly is caused by a somatotroph pituitary tumour secreting growth hormone (GH) in 95% of cases, but may also be caused by tumours secreting growth hormone releasing hormone (GHRH), e.g. carcinoid tumours, pancreatic islet cell tumours, small cell carcinoma of the lung and medullary carcinoma of the thyroid.

Hypoglycaemia is a potent stimulus for GH release and, conversely, an acute rise in the blood sugar inhibits GH release. The failure of GH levels to suppress after an oral glucose load is characteristic of acromegaly and is the diagnostic test most frequently employed. In acromegaly there is an exaggerated GH response to insulin-induced hypoglycaemia and to an arginine infusion test. The IGF-1 (somatomedin-C) concentration is a useful screening test for acromegaly and can be used to monitor treatment. Hypercalciuria is a frequent finding and is due to increased circulating dihydroxyvitamin D. The presence of hypercalcaemia in a patient with acromegaly suggests primary hyperparathyroidism because of the multiple endocrine neoplasia type I syndrome (MEN I; Wermer's syndrome).

3.21 (a) T (b) F (c) F (d) T (e) F

Porphyrias are inherited diseases characterized by deficiencies of enzymes involved in porphyrin synthesis. As a result of these deficiencies there is increased activity of ALA synthase, leading to excessive production of porphyrins or their precursors. Diseases which result in increased production of porphyrin precursors (ALA and PBG) have neurological complications, while those diseases resulting in increased porphyrin synthesis develop photosensitivity. Porphyrias may either be classified as acute and non-acute, or as hepatic and erythropoietic (Table 3.4).

Table 3.4 Biochemical features of porphyrias

Porphyria	Enzyme defect	↑ in urine	↑ in stool
Acute, intermittent*†	Porphobilinogen deaminase	ALA, PBG	–
Variegate porphyria*†	Protoporphyrinogen oxidase	ALA, PBG, coproporphyrinogen	Coproporphyrinogen, protoporphyrinogen
Hereditary coproporphyria*†	Coproporphyrinogen oxidase	ALA, PBG, coproporphyrinogen	Coproporphyrinogen
Porphyria cutanea tarda§†	Uroporphyrinogen decarboxylase	Uroporphyrinogen	Isocoproporphyrinogen
Congenital erythropoietic porphyria§‡	Uroporphyrinogen III cosynthase	Uroporphyrinogen, coproporphyrinogen	Coproporphyrinogen
Erythropoietic protoporphyria§‡	Ferrochelatase	–	Protoporphyrinogen

*Acute, † hepatic, ‡ erythropoietic, § non-acute.

3.22 (a) F (b) T (c) F (d) T (e) T

ANCA may be positive in a number of diseases characterized by systemic necrotizing vasculitis and are often of value in monitoring disease activity. Indirect immunofluorescence shows two patterns of staining: cytoplasmic (c-ANCA) and perinuclear (p-ANCA). The c-ANCA is 88% sensitive and 95% specific for Wegener's granulomatosis, but may also be found in idiopathic crescentic glomerulonephritis, and in some cases of microscopic polyarteritis. The major c-ANCA antigen is proteinase 3 (PR3), a 29 kDa serine protease in neutrophil azurophilic granules. The majority of p-ANCA are directed towards myeloperoxidase (MPO), but other target antigens may include elastase, lactoferrin and cathepsin G. About 75% of patients with microscopic polyarteritis are positive for p-ANCA (directed towards MPO). The presence of p-ANCA has also been described in Churg–Strauss syndrome, polyarteritis nodosa, ulcerative colitis and primary sclerosing cholangitis. In rare cases, p-ANCA may be associated with systemic lupus erythematosus, rheumatoid arthritis and Henoch–Schönlein purpura. Recently, an ANCA directed towards a neutrophil endotoxin-binding protein has been described. The bactericidal/permeability increasing protein ANCA (BPI-ANCA) has been described in association with ulcerative colitis, primary sclerosing cholangitis and cystic fibrosis.

3.23 (a) F (b) T (c) T (d) T (e) F

Calcium and phosphate homeostasis are controlled through several hormone systems. PTH is secreted in response to low plasma calcium concentrations. The overall effect of PTH is to increase plasma calcium and decrease phosphate. PTH stimulates increased renal reabsorption of calcium and increased calcium absorption from the gut. PTH also promotes calcium resorption from bone and stimulates increased synthesis of 1,25-dihydroxycholecalciferol (1,25$(OH)_2$D) by the proximal convoluted tubule. PTH increases renal excretion of inorganic phosphate. Calcitonin, a peptide hormone secreted by the C cells of the thyroid gland, inhibits calcium resorption from bone and increases renal excretion of phosphate. The precise biological role of calcitonin is unclear, since patients with medullary carcinoma of the thyroid have excess calcitonin but never exhibit symptoms of hypocalcaemia; conversely, calcitonin supplementation is not required after thyroidectomy and patients never exhibit signs of hypercalcaemia. Vitamin D is a hormone synthesized from 7-dehydrocholesterol (provitamin D_3). The action of ultraviolet light on the skin converts provitamin D_3 to vitamin D_3. This is hydroxylated in the liver to 25-hydroxycholecalciferol (25(OH)D). The final step in the formation of the active hormone occurs in the kidney, where renal mitochondrial 25(OH)D-1α-hydroxylase hydroxylates either the C_1 or C_{24} position to produce 1,25$(OH)_2$D and 24,25$(OH)_2$D, respectively. However, 1,25$(OH)_2$D is the only active metabolite of vitamin D.

3.24 (a) T (b) F (c) F (d) T (e) T

Respiratory alkalosis is the earliest acid–base disturbance in acute salicylate poisoning, and is due to direct stimulation of the respiratory centre by salicylate. Consequently, there is increased urinary excretion of bicarbonate, sodium, potassium and water; and therefore hyponatremia, hypokalaemia and passage of alkaline urine are typical of early poisoning. Dehydration results from vomiting, pyrexia and hyperventilation, sometimes leading to acute renal failure. Salicylate uncouples oxidative phosphorylation, resulting in accumulation of lactate and pyruvate. Other features of late salicylate poisoning including increased lipolysis with ketone formation, and accelerated proteolysis leading to aminoaciduria. Elevated haematocrit, elevated platelet count, hypernatremia, hyperkalaemia, hypoglycaemia, abnormal liver function tests and prolonged prothrombin time may also be seen. Tinnitus occurs at low concentrations of salicylate, and may even occur when salicylate levels are within the therapeutic range.

3.25 (a) T (b) F (c) F (d) T (e) T

The Haemoccult card consists of a filter paper impregnated with gum guaiac. A faecal sample is smeared onto the paper and a developer solution of hydrogen peroxide is added. Haemoglobin has peroxidase-like activity which changes the test paper blue. Dietary sources of haemoglobin, myoglobin and other oxidants may affect the test: patients should be asked to avoid eating meat, fresh fruit, some vegetables (cauliflower, swede, turnip, tomatoes, horseradish) and vitamin C supplements for 3 days before testing. Aspirin and other non-steroidals should be avoided as they may increase blood loss through gastrointestinal irritation. Ferrous sulphate does not affect the guaiac test. Normal daily blood loss from the gastrointestinal tract is 0.5–1.2 ml. Daily blood loss must exceed 20 ml for a reliable result with the Haemoccult system. As a screening tool, the sensitivity of the test is limited because most colonic tumours bleed intermittently; carcinomas are more likely to bleed than adenomas. Screening studies have shown that occult blood testing will miss some 40% of colonic cancers, and about 80% of larger adenomas. The Haemoccult test is more sensitive for left-sided tumours than for right-sided and rectal tumours. This apparent paradox may be because the test relies on the release of haematin from degraded haemoglobin: fresh blood from distal tumours may be insufficiently haemolysed. The sensitivity of the test can be increased by rehydrating the test paper with a drop of water before testing – this may facilitate lysis of red blood cells and the release and degradation of haemoglobin. However, this decreases specificity, and is not generally advised.

FURTHER READING

Leaker, B. and Cambridge, G. (1993) Clinical use of anti-neutrophil cytoplasmic antibodies, *Br J Hosp Med*, **50**, 540–7.

Marshall, W.J. (1995) *Clinical Chemistry*, 3rd edn, Mosby, London.

Mulcahy, H.E., Farthing, M.J.G. and O'Donoghue, D.P. (1997) Screening for asymptomatic colorectal cancer, *BMJ*, **314**, 285–91.

Stoffel, M.P., Csernok, C., Herzber, T. *et al.* (1996) Anti-neutrophil cytoplasmic antibodies (ANCA) directed against bactericidal permeability increasing protein (BPI): a new seromarker for inflammatory bowel disease and associated disorders. *Clin Exp Immunol*, **104**, 54–9.

4 Haematology and immunology

QUESTIONS

4.1 The following statements are true:

(a) haemoglobin has a molecular weight of approximately 64 000.
(b) haem is formed by the addition of Fe^{3+} to protoporphyrin IX.
(c) the gene for the α-globin chain is located on chromosome 16.
(d) 50% of a normal adult's haemoglobin is in the form of haemoglobin A.
(e) levels of foetal haemoglobin (HbF) may be raised in sickle cell disease.

4.2 The following haemoglobin (Hb) concentrations may be regarded as normal:

(a) Hb 18 g/dl in a neonate.
(b) Hb 9 g/dl in a 3-month old baby.
(c) Hb 9 g/dl in a 10-year old child.
(d) Hb 13 g/dl in an adult male.
(e) Hb 18 g/dl in an adult female.

4.3 Erythrocytes:

(a) have a life span of approximately 120 days in the circulation.
(b) express HLA class II antigens on the cell surface.
(c) do not contain mitochondria.
(d) are released into the circulation from the bone marrow as mature erythrocytes.
(e) in hereditary spherocytosis have an abnormality of the spectrin molecule of the cytoskeleton.

4.4 The following statements are true:

(a) Howell Jolly bodies are a feature of glucose-6-phosphate dehydrogenase (G6PD) deficiency.
(b) Heinz bodies are a feature of haemolytic anaemia.
(c) acanthocytosis may be a feature of hypothyroidism.
(d) spherocytes may be seen in the blood film of patients with severe burns.
(e) Burr cells are a recognized feature of uraemia.

4.5 The following are recognized causes of macrocytosis on the peripheral blood film with a normoblastic bone marrow:
(a) jejunal diverticulosis.
(b) hypothyroidism.
(c) pregnancy.
(d) phenytoin.
(e) zidovudine.

4.6 The following statements regarding platelets are true:
(a) platelets have a life span of approximately 28 days.
(b) platelets express HLA class I antigen on their surface.
(c) platelets contain mitochondria.
(d) thromboxane A_2 potentiates platelet aggregation.
(e) prostacyclin (PGI_2) is a potent inhibitor of platelet aggregation.

4.7 The following statements regarding the coagulation cascade are true:
(a) the extrinsic pathway is initiated by collagen exposure.
(b) ristocetin-induced platelet activation is dependent on factor VIII.
(c) factor Xa converts prothrombin to thrombin.
(d) fibrin cross-linkage is catalysed by factor XII.
(e) plasmin inactivates factors V and VIII.

4.8 Regarding neutrophils:
(a) the nucleus usually consists of eight segments.
(b) life span in the circulation is approximately 10 hours.
(c) they have surface receptors for the Fab fragment of immunoglobulin G (IgG).
(d) Auer rods may be a feature of acute myeloid leukaemia.
(e) the ability to phagocytose bacteria is impaired in chronic granulomatous disease.

4.9 Basophilia is a recognized feature of:
(a) chronic myeloid leukaemia.
(b) hypothyroidism.
(c) dermatitis herpetiformis.
(d) ulcerative colitis.
(e) Cushing's syndrome.

4.10 The following statements regarding eosinophils are correct:
(a) eosinophils are phagocytes.
(b) eosinophils are essential to the host defence against bacterial infection.
(c) cytoplasmic granules principally contain histamine.
(d) eosinophil chemotactic factor of anaphylaxis (ECFa) is derived from mast cells.
(e) glucocorticoid therapy may induce eosinopenia.

4.11 The following statements regarding lymphocytes are true:
(a) B cells represent 70% of circulating lymphocytes.
(b) B lymphocytes are the predominant cell type in the paracortical region of the lymph node.
(c) T lymphocytes form rosettes when centrifuged with sheep erythrocytes.
(d) T lymphocytes do not express surface immunoglobulin G (IgG).
(e) CD3 receptors are found on the surface of all T lymphocytes.

4.12 T lymphocytes:
(a) undergo differentiation in the thymus.
(b) all possess the T cell surface receptor (TCR).
(c) may enter lymph nodes through high endothelial venules.
(d) are important in the initiation of the secondary immune response.
(e) have an important role in contact dermatitis.

4.13 The following are recognized antigen-presenting cells:
(a) neutrophils.
(b) mast cells.
(c) macrophages.
(d) B lymphocytes.
(e) Langerhans cells.

4.14 The major histocompatibility complex (MHC):
(a) is located on chromosome 6.
(b) class I antigens are expressed on the surface of all nucleated cells.
(c) class II antigens include the series DP, DQ and DR.
(d) $CD4^+$ cells only recognize antigen when presented in association with MHC class II molecules.
(e) MHC antigen matching significantly improves the outcome of organ transplantation.

4.15 The Fc region of the immunoglobulin molecule determines:
(a) antibody specificity.
(b) ability for transplacental transfer.
(c) the half-life of the immunoglobulin molecule.
(d) mast cell binding.
(e) activation of the complement cascade.

4.16 Immunoglobulin G (IgG)
(a) has a molecular weight of 400 000 kDa.
(b) is able to cross the placenta.
(c) constitutes the rheumatoid factor.
(d) is the principal immunoglobulin in bronchial secretions.
(e) activates complement via the classical pathway.

4.17 Secretory immunoglobulin A (sIgA):
(a) is a pentamer.
(b) crosses the placental barrier.
(c) is responsible for mucosal immunity.
(d) activates the classical complement pathway.
(e) is synthesized by plasma cells in regional lymph nodes.

4.18 The following statements are correct:
(a) the classical pathway is activated by C1q binding to the Fab fragment of immunoglobulin M (IgM).
(b) bacterial endotoxin activates the alternative pathway.
(c) C2 is activated via both classical and alternative pathways.
(d) C5a is a potent neutrophil chemotactic agent.
(e) individuals with a deficiency of C5 are at increased risk of developing meningococcal septicaemia.

4.19 Type I hypersensitivity reactions:
(a) typically evolve over a period of days.
(b) occur when an immunoglobulin E-antigen complex binds to the surface of a mast cell.
(c) are responsible for the 'weal and flare' response.
(d) may be prevented by therapeutic use of sodium cromoglycate.
(e) are responsible for serum sickness.

4.20 Type IV (delayed) hypersensitivity responses:
(a) do not involve activation of complement.
(b) are mediated primarily through a T_H2 response.
(c) typically develop within 72 h of exposure to the antigen.
(d) form the basis of the Heaf test.
(e) are the cause of contact dermatitis.

4.21 Interferons:
(a) play an important role in host defence against bacteria.
(b) are synthesized by B lymphocytes.
(c) have an inhibitory effect on granulocyte and macrophage killing.
(d) have anti-tumour activity.
(e) in the form of gamma interferon (γIFN) may be used in the treatment of chronic hepatitis C infection.

4.22 Regarding interleukins (IL):
(a) IL-1 is an endogenous pyrogen.
(b) IL-2 is produced principally by CD4+ T cells.
(c) IL-3 stimulates growth of all haemopoietic precursors.
(d) IL-4 inhibits production of inflammatory cytokines.
(e) IL-6 stimulates hepatic production of acute phase proteins.

4.23 An acute phase response:
(a) is associated with increased tumour necrosis factor production.
(b) is accompanied by a rise in the serum iron level.
(c) may induce a fever.
(d) is easily monitored by measuring C3b levels.
(e) to viral infection is more marked than the response to bacterial infection.

4.24 The following statements are true:
(a) the natural haemagglutinins (anti-A and anti-B) are of immunoglobulin M (IgM) type.
(b) anti-D antibody is non-agglutinating.
(c) type AB blood should not be transfused to type O recipients.
(d) anti-I antibodies may develop following *Mycoplasma pneumoniae* infection.
(e) carcinoma of the stomach is commoner in individuals with blood group A.

4.25 Regarding transplant immunology:
(a) matching for HLA class II antigens is more important than matching for class I antigens in determining graft survival in renal transplantation.
(b) HLA matching is not required for cardiac transplantation.
(c) acute rejection may occur up to 3 months after transplantation.
(d) patients who have received multiple blood transfusions before renal transplantation are at increased risk of subsequent graft rejection.
(e) T cell depletion of donor bone marrow reduces the incidence of graft *versus* host disease.

ANSWERS

4.1 (a) T (b) F (c) T (d) F (e) T

Haemoglobin is a tetrameric protein with a molecular weight of approximately 64 000. It is composed of two pairs of polypeptides (e.g. $\alpha_2\beta_2$), each covalently linked to a haem moiety. Haem is formed by the addition of ferrous iron (Fe^{2+}) to protoporphyrin IX. The gene for a α-globin is located on chromosome 16. The genes for the β, δ and γ sub-units are located on chromosome 11. Of a normal adult's haemoglobin, 90% is in the form of HbA ($\alpha_2\beta_2$). Haemoglobin A2 concentration is increased in β thalassaemia. Haemoglobin F ($\alpha_2\gamma_2$) is the main haemoglobin component in foetal erythrocytes: synthesis of γ-chains switches to synthesis of β-chains during the third trimester. Production of γ-chains persists in β thalassaemia and in sickle cell disease. The α and β thalassaemias are characterized by imbalance in globin chain synthesis.

4.2 (a) T (b) F (c) F (d) T (e) F

Age	**Haemoglobin concentration**
Neonate (1–3 days)	13–21 g/dl
<1 month	10–18 g/dl
1–12 months	10–13.5 g/dl
1–12 years	11.5–15.5 g/dl
Adult male	13–18 g/dl
Adult female	12–16 g/dl

4.3 (a) T (b) F (c) T (d) F (e) T

Newly formed reticulocytes remain in the bone marrow for 2–3 days before being released into the circulation, and subsequently lose their mitochondria and ribosomes to become mature erythrocytes. The mature erythrocyte is a flexible biconcave disc, measuring 8 μm in diameter. The lifespan is approximately 120 days (measured by ^{51}Cr labelling). Four major proteins (spectrin, actin, protein 4.1 and ankyrin) form a mesh on the inner aspect of the cell membrane and are important in maintaining the shape and flexibility of the cell. Defects in the membrane components explain some morphological abnormalities: hereditary spherocytosis is caused by an abnormality in the spectrin molecule; a large increase in the cholesterol content of the red blood cell membrane may cause acanthocytosis; and increases in phospholipid and cholesterol in the membrane may be responsible for target cell formation. HLA class II antigens are expressed only on the surface of activated T cells, B cells, macrophages and damaged endothelium.

4.4 (a) F (b) F (c) T (d) T (e) T

Heinz bodies are precipitates of haemoglobin or globin sub-units, and are seen in unstable forms of haemoglobin (e.g. Hb Hammersmith, HbS, HbC and HbD), thalassaemia, oxidant drugs and in G6PD deficiency.

Howell Jolly bodies and **Cabot's rings** are remnants of nuclear material seen in megaloblastic anaemia and hyposplenism, particularly following splenectomy. Iron granules (siderocytes) are also a frequent finding after splenectomy.

Acanthocytes are seen in abetalipoproteinaemia, and other disorders of lipid metabolism. They may be a feature of hypothyroidism, severe anorexia nervosa and alcoholic liver disease.

Spherocytosis may be hereditary or acquired. Genetic causes include hereditary spherocytosis and HbC disease. Acquired causes include Coombs' positive autoimmune haemolytic anaemias and severe burns (damaged red blood cell membranes).

Basophilic stippling indicates either accelerated erythropoiesis or defective haemoglobin synthesis and is characteristically seen in lead poisoning.

Burr cells (echinocytes) are regularly crenated, scalloped erythrocytes and are common artifacts on the blood film. They are also seen in uraemia and pyruvate kinase deficiency.

4.5 (a) F (b) T (c) T (d) F (e) T

Conditions, other than vitamin B_{12} and folate deficiency, which cause a macrocytosis include:

1. pregnancy;
2. endocrine: hypothyroidism;
3. respiratory: chronic respiratory failure;
4. haematological: acquired sideroblastic anaemia, myelodysplastic syndromes, leukoerythroblastic anaemia, multiple myeloma and reticulocytosis (haemolytic anaemia, acute haemorrhage);
5. hepatic: chronic liver disease and alcoholism. The commonest cause of a raised mean corpuscular volume is alcohol. This can occur without anaemia and with a normoblastic marrow, but can also be because of dietary folate deficiency or a direct toxic effect of alcohol on the bone marrow;
6. abnormalities of B_{12} or folate metabolism: transcobalamin II deficiency, homocystinuria, nitrous oxide and dihydrofolate reductase inhibitors (methotrexate, pyrimethamine and trimethoprim);
7. defects of DNA synthesis independent of B_{12} and folate: orotic aciduria, Lesch–Nyhan syndrome, acquired sideroblastic anaemia, drugs inhibiting purine or pyrimidine synthesis (zidovudine (AZT),

hydroxyurea, 6-mercaptopurine, cytosine, arabinoside and 5-fluorouracil) and alcohol. In each of these conditions the bone marrow is normal and neutrophils are not hypersegmented.

Hypersegmented neutrophils (six lobes or more) are associated with vitamin B_{12} and folate deficiency. Jejunal diverticulosis and phenytoin therapy are associated with vitamin B_{12} deficiency.

4.6 (a) F (b) T (c) T (d) T (e) T

Platelets are disc-shaped cells measuring 1–2 μm in diameter, synthesized in the bone marrow from megakaryocytes. Normal platelet life span is 7–10 days. The bilamellar cell membrane is composed of glycoproteins and phospholipids. These glycoproteins are important for platelet adhesion and aggregation: glycoproteins Ia and IIa facilitate adhesion to collagen; glycoprotein Ib binds von Willebrand factor and is defective in Bernard–Soulier disease; glycoproteins IIb and IIIa bind fibrinogen; glycoprotein V is the thrombin receptor. Membrane phosphilipids (platelet factor 3) are necessary for the conversion of coagulation factor X to Xa and for the conversion of prothrombin to thrombin. Antigens expressed on the platelet surface include ABO and HLA class I antigens.

Platelets contain mitochondria, lysosomes, a dense tubular system, and two types of granule. Electron-dense granules contain ADP, calcium and serotonin. The α-granules contain platelet-derived growth factor (PDGF), fibrinogen, factor V, von Willebrand factor, fibronectin, platelet factor 4 (heparin antagonist), thrombospondin and β-thromboglobulin. Prostaglandins and thromboxane A_2 are synthesized in the tubular system. Platelets do not have a nucleus. Prostacyclin (PGI_2) is synthesized by vascular endothelial cells.

4.7 (a) F (b) T (c) T (d) F (e) T (Figure 4.1)

4.8 (a) F (b) T (c) F (d) T (e) F

Neutrophils (polymorphs) are mobile phagocytic cells produced in the bone marrow. Maturation of neutrophil progenitor cells is influenced by granulocyte-colony stimulating factor (G-CSF). Neutrophils have receptors for C3b and for the Fc portion of IgG, which facilitate opsonization of foreign particles. The normal count is 2.5–7.5 × 10^9/l. The mature neutrophil nucleus usually contains up to five segments: hypersegmentation is a feature of vitamin B_{12} or folate deficiency. Bilobed nuclei are seen in the Pelger–Huët anomaly (due to failure of nuclear segmentation): this may be inherited as a benign autosomal dominant trait, but is also seen in leukaemias or infection. Döhle bodies are cytoplasmic inclusion bodies seen during acute infection,

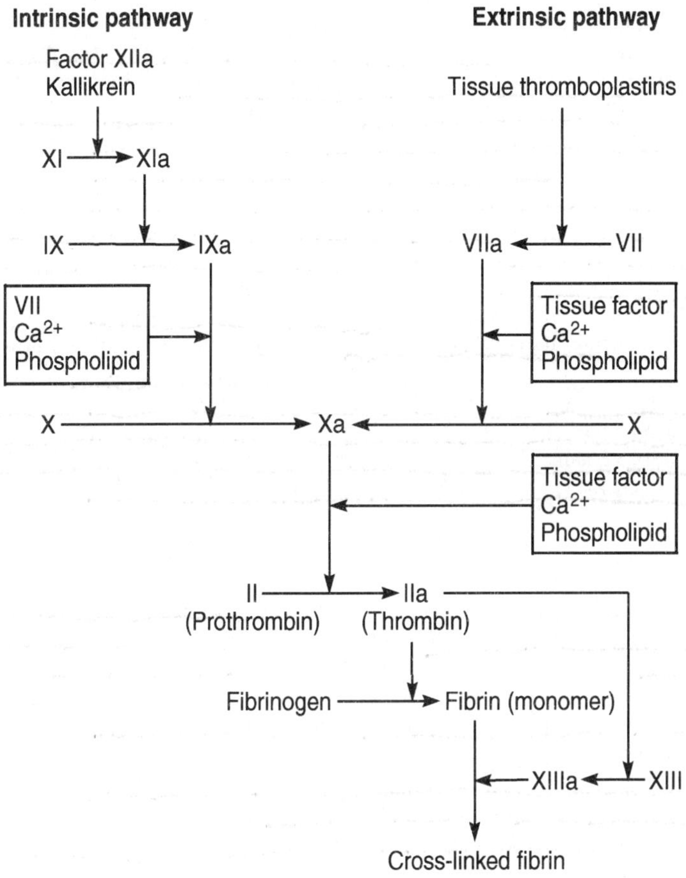

Figure 4.1 Coagulation cascade.

pregnancy, malignancy, trauma and after cytotoxic chemotherapy. Auer rods are cytoplasmic inclusions seen in myeloblasts and promyelocytes of some patients with acute myeloid leukaemia.

Hydrogen peroxide, superoxide and other oxygen radicals are produced in cytoplasmic granules. After phagocytosis, these granules fuse with the phagocytic vacuole. In chronic granulomatous disease phagocytosis is normal, but neutrophils are unable to kill bacteria because of a defect in oxidative metabolism.

4.9 (a) T (b) T (c) F (d) T (e) F

Basophils are only occasionally seen in the peripheral blood and constitute less than 1% of the total leukocyte count. Their cytoplasm contains darkly staining granules which contain heparin, histamine and eosinophil chemotactic factor of anaphylaxis (ECFa). Basophils are involved in immediate (type I) hypersensitivity reactions and have surface receptors for the Fc portion of IgE and for activated complement components (C3a, C5a). Degranulation is associated with histamine release, resulting in smooth muscle contraction and increased vascular permeability. The normal count is less than $0.1 \times 10^9/l$.

Basophilia is associated with myeloproliferative disorders, particularly chronic myeloid leukaemia and myelosclerosis. Less marked increases in the peripheral basophil count occur in hypothyroidism, ulcerative colitis, tuberculosis, haemolytic anaemias, cancers and after splenectomy. Dermatitis herpetiformis may be associated with an eosinophilia; Cushing's syndrome is associated with eosinopenia, but was described by Harvey Cushing in 1932 as 'pituitary basophilia'.

4.10 (a) T (b) F (c) F (d) T (e) T

Eosinophils are characterized by their large cytoplasmic granules which stain red with eosin. These granules contain a strongly basic protein, the major basic protein, capable of neutralizing heparin, and eosinophil peroxidase. Eosinophil cytoplasm contains cationic proteins, Charcot–Leyden crystals and a potent neurotoxin. Although eosinophils and neutrophils share similar morphology and function (surface receptors for immunoglobulin G, chemotactic responses, phagocytic capacity and lysosomal enzymes), the main role of eosinophils is in eliminating parasites and participation in hypersensitivity reactions. The normal count is $0.04–0.4 \times 10^9/l$.

Causes of eosinophilia $> 0.4 \times 10^9/l$ are as follows:

1. allergic disorders: asthma, hay fever, food allergy, serum sickness and drug reactions;
2. parasitic infections (particularly helminthic infections);
3. skin disorders: eczema, urticaria, psoriasis, pemphigus and dermatitis herpetiformis;
4. malignancies: Hodgkin's lymphoma, mycosis fungoides, chronic myeloid leukaemia, melanoma and carcinomas (lung, pancreas, stomach, ovary and uterus);
5. hypereosinophilic syndromes: Loeffler's syndrome, eosinophilic leukaemia and idiopathic hypereosinophilic syndrome;
6. miscellaneous: polyarteritis nodosa, ulcerative colitis, sarcoidosis, hypoadrenalism and chronic granulomatous disease.

Eosinopenia occurs with stress, after acute bacterial infections and after administration of glucocorticoids.

4.11 (a) F (b) F (c) T (d) T (e) T

Lymphocytes represent approximately 20% of the total leukocyte count. B cells undergo maturation in the bone marrow, while T cell differentiation occurs in the thymus. In lymph nodes, T cells occupy the paracortical areas surrounding the germinal centres; B cells are located within primary and secondary lymphoid follicles, and within germinal centres and in the spleen. In the spleen, T cells occupy the periarteriolar areas of white pulp; B cells occupy the follicular zone (containing germinal centres) and the marginal zone of the white pulp. T cells constitute 70% of the circulating lymphocyte population and are the principal effectors of the cell-mediated immune response. T cells are capable of binding sheep erythrocytes by means of the CD2 surface receptor. Mature B cells comprise 10–15% of the peripheral blood lymphocytes. B cells, but not T cells, express surface IgG. The primary function of B cells is to produce antibodies.

The cluster designation (CD) system indicates specific cell marker molecules which can be identified by monoclonal antibody staining. These include the integrins, selectins, proteoglycans (CD44), and the immunoglobulin superfamily (including CD2, CD3, CD4 and CD8), so named because of their structural similarity to immunoglobulin molecules.

4.12 (a) T (b) T (c) T (d) T (e) T

The definitive T cell marker is the T cell antigen receptor (TCR), a two-chain molecule resembling the immunoglobulin molecule. Two types of TCR have been identified to date: TCRα/β consists of α and β sub-units; TCRδ/γ is composed of δ and γ polypeptide sub-units. Both are associated with CD3 to form the TCR–CD3 complex. Most T cells (90%) express TCRα/β. The CD4 molecule is found on helper T lymphocytes (T_H), and is the receptor for the human immunodeficiency virus (HIV). CD8 is found on cytotoxic T cells (T_C). The secondary immune response is initiated by memory T and B cells following a further exposure to the same antigen.

Lymphocytes may enter lymph nodes through afferent lymphatics, or via high endothelial venules in the paracortical T cell areas. These structures are absent from the spleen, bone marrow and thymus.

4.13 (a) F (b) F (c) T (d) T (e) T

Antigen presenting cells (APCs) are located mainly in the spleen, lymph nodes, skin and thymus. The APCs in the skin are the Langerhans cells of the epidermis which are capable of migration, as 'veiled' cells, to the paracortical ares of local lymph nodes where they interact with T_H cells. Follicular dendritic cells in the secondary follicles and germinal centres of lymph nodes are responsible for antigen presentation to B cells. Follicular dendritic cells do not express the major histocompatibility complex (MHC) class II molecule. Other APCs include macrophages, B cells and interdigitating medullary cells in the thymus. Endothelial or epithelial cells may acquire the ability to present antigens when induced by cytokines such as tumour necrosis factor alpha (TNFα) and interferon gamma (IFNγ).

Antigen must be presented along with an MHC molecule for antigen recognition by lymphocytes: T_H cells (CD4+) only recognize APCs bearing MHC class II, whereas T_C (CD8+) only recognize those APCs bearing MHC class I molecules. APCs secrete interleukin-1 (IL-1), inducing clonal T cell proliferation, but IL-2 (produced by T_H cells) is also required.

4.14 (a) T (b) T (c) T (d) T (e) T

The major histocompatibility complex (MHC), located on the short arm of chromosome 6, is responsible for cell–cell interactions in the adaptive immune system. The gene products of the MHC in man are called the human leukocyte antigens (HLA). These genes lie in three groups known as classes I, II and III. Accurate HLA matches are essential to minimize the risk of graft *versus* host disease after bone marrow transplantation, and are also important in minimizing rejection of solid organ transplants.

Class I antigens have alleles at the A, B and C loci and are expressed on the surface of all nucleated cells. Class I molecules are heterodimers composed of a heavy (α) chain and β_2 microglobulin (a polypeptide encoded on chromosome 12). Variations in the class I molecules are due to differences in the heavy chain, while the β_2 microglobulin component remains constant. HLA class I antigens are mainly concerned with recognition of viral antigen by cytotoxic (CD8+) lymphocytes.

Class II antigens resemble the T cell receptor. They are composed of a heavy (α) and light (β) chain and include the antigens DP, DQ and DR. They have a restricted distribution confined to B cells, activated T cells, macrophages, inflamed vascular endothelium and some epithelial cells. Interferon gamma is able to induce expression of class II antigens on some cells (thyroid, pancreas and gut epithelium) in response to inflammation. HLA class II molecules are essential for antigen recognition by T helper (CD4+) cells.

Class III MHC antigens include some components of the complement pathway (C2, C4 and Factor B), but are functionally unrelated to class I and II molecules.

4.15 (a) F (b) T (c) T (d) T (e) T
All immunoglobulins have a basic structure composed of two heavy and two light chains. Light chains may be either kappa (κ) or lambda (λ). Each immunoglobulin is determined by the type of heavy chain present. The light chains each have one variable and one constant region; the heavy chains one variable unit and three or four constant units. Papain, a protease enzyme, cleaves the immunoglobulin molecule at the hinge region into two separate fragments – the Fab (antibody binding) and Fc (crystallizable) fragments. The Fc fragment determines the effector functions of the immunoglobulin molecule: complement fixation, monocyte and macrophage binding, control of breakdown and transplacental transfer. The Fab fragment is contained within the variable regions VL and VH. Within these variable domains are the six hypervariable regions which determine the antibody's specificity.

4.16 (a) F (b) T (c) F (d) F (e) T
(See answer 4.17)

4.17 (a) F (b) F (c) T (d) F (e) F
IgG (molecular weight 150 000) is the major immunoglobulin in the serum, constituting 70–75% of the total immunoglobulin pool, and is the principal immunoglobulin of the secondary immune response. In humans IgG is the only immunoglobulin capable of crossing the placental barrier, and does so in an active process involving specific placental receptors for the Fc fragment. This confers immunity in neonates, but transplacental transfer of IgG is also responsible for autoimmune disease in the neonate: Grave's disease, myasthenia gravis and congenital heart block in systemic lupus erythematosus (mother anti-Ro (SS-A) positive). IgG_1 and IgG_3 are the most effective opsonins and activators of complement.

IgA constitutes 15–20% of the total serum immunoglobulin pool, more than 80% existing in the monomeric (IgA_1) form (molecular weight 160 000). IgA_2 is the principal immunoglobulin in secretions (saliva, tears, milk, colostrum, gastrointestinal and bronchial secrétions). Secretory IgA (sIgA) exists mainly in the dimeric (molecular weight 320 000) form in these secretions. Plasma cells in mucosa-associated lymphoid tissue (MALT) synthesize monomeric IgA which is dimerized by the addition of a joining ('J') piece. Epithelial cells

Table 4.1 Properties of immunoglobulins

Class	Subclass	Heavy chains	Molecular weight	Plasma level (g/l)	% Total Ig level	Classical pathway	Alternative pathway	Cells bound *via* Fc receptor
IgG	IgG_1	γ_1	150 000	9	70–75	√	×	Macrophages, neutrophils, eosinophils, large granular lymphocytes
	IgG_2	γ_2	150 000	3		√	×	
	IgG_3	γ_3	170 000	1		√	×	
	IgG_4	γ_4	150 000	0.5 (Total 8–19)		×	√	
IgA	IgA_1	α_1	160 000 (monomer)	3	15–20	×	√	Lymphocytes
	IgA_2	α_2	320 000 (dimer)	0.5 (Total 1.4–4.0)		×		
IgM		μ	970 000 (pentamer)	0.5–2.0	10	√	×	Lymphocytes
IgD		δ	170 000	30×10^{-3}	<1	×	√	None
IgE		ε	185 000	$0–50 \times 10^{-9}$	<<1	×	√	Mast cells, basophils, B cells

synthesize a glycopeptide, the secretory piece, which acts as a cellular receptor for the sIgA molecule, which is transported across the mucosa and into the intestinal lumen. The secretory piece also prevents digestion of the IgA molecule by proteolytic enzymes.

The **IgM** molecule is a pentamer of molecular weight 900 000, constituting approximately 10% of the immunoglobulin pool. IgM is largely confined to the blood and is the first antibody to be produced in the primary immune response. It is very effective at fixing complement. The blood group antigens (natural haemagglutinins) are of the IgM class. Rheumatoid factor is IgM directed against IgG.

IgD is mainly located on the surface of B cells, and is present only in small quantities in the plasma.

IgE is found in very small amounts in the plasma and is mainly bound to the surface of mast cells, bound by the Fc region. Cross-binding of IgE molecules on the surface of mast cells and basophils leads to degranulation and release of inflammatory mediators.

Further information about immunoglobulins is given in Table 4.1.

4.18 (a) F (b) T (c) F (d) T (e) T

The three main functions of complement are: (1) opsonization of antigen, binding the target for phagocytosis, (2) activation of polymorphs and macrophages, and (3) lysis, by insertion of a membrane attack complex through the target cell membrane. The **classical pathway** is activated by antibody–antigen complexes, and therefore works in conjunction with the adaptive immune system. C1 is the first enzyme complex in this cascade, which binds the Fc fragment of immunoglobulin via its C1q component. Further steps involve C2, C4 and C3. The **alternative pathway** does not rely on antibody – bacterial cell walls and endotoxin are the most potent stimuli to activation. Interaction of the glycoprotein properdin, the proteins factor B and factor D, and C3b generate C3 convertase. Both pathways converge at C3 to form the final lytic pathway by forming the membrane attack complex (C5–9).

C3a and C5a are anaphylotoxins, causing vasodilatation and increasing vascular permeability, thereby facilitating the movement of other components of the immune response to the site of inflammation. C5a is a potent neutrophil chemotactic agent which promotes phagocytosis by upgrading CR1 and CR3 receptors on neutrophils. C3a, also a chemotaxin, is much less potent than C5a. All of these small peptides have a very short half-life.

Deficiencies of classical pathway components predispose to recurrent pyogenic bacterial infections. Deficiencies of elements of the membrane attack complex (C5–9) result in increased susceptibility to infection with *Neisseria meningitidis*.

4.19 (a) F (b) F (c) T (d) T (e) F

Type I (immediate or anaphylactic) hypersensitivity occurs when mast cells degranulate in response to an antigenic stimulus. IgE is present on the mast cell surface, bound by its Fc fragment. On contact with the appropriate allergen the IgE molecules cross-link, causing degranulation and release of preformed inflammatory mediators which include chemoattractants (cytokines e.g. IL-5, IL-8 and TNF), vasodilators (kinins and histamine) and spasmogens (histamine causes bronchial smooth muscle contraction). This reaction is rapid: when the appropriate antigen is injected into the skin a typical 'weal and flare' response can be seen within 5–10 min. Examples of type I reactions include anaphylactic reactions to bee stings, hay fever (antigen: pollen), and asthma (antigen: house dust mite). Sodium cromoglycate stabilizes the mast cell membrane.

Serum sickness is an example of a type III (immune complex) hypersensitivity reaction. **Type III (Arthus) responses** occur when circulating antibody–antigen complexes become deposited in the tissues. These immune complexes activate complement and tissue damage results from the ensuing inflammatory response. Immune complex diseases can be because of persistent infection (leprosy, viral hepatitis, malaria or post-streptococcal glomerulonephritis), autoimmune disease (rheumatoid arthritis, systemic lupus erythematosus, Henoch-Schönlein purpura or mixed cryoglobulinaemia), or diseases caused by inhaled antigen (extrinsic allergic alveolitis, where type IV hypersensitivity also plays an important role).

4.20 (a) T (b) F (c) T (d) T (e) T

Type IV (cell-mediated or delayed) hypersensitivity is mediated through antigen-specific T cells. The three main varieties of type IV reactions include contact (contact dermatitis), tuberculin (Heaf test), and granulomatous (Kveim test) responses. Contact and tuberculin hypersensitivity reactions develop within 72 h of exposure to antigen; granulomatous reactions take place over 21–28 days. Diseases that manifest type IV hypersensitivity reactions include leprosy (particularly the borderline type), tuberculosis, sarcoidosis, Crohn's disease, extrinsic allergic alveolitis, graft *versus* host disease, acute graft rejection, and schistosomiasis.

Two subsets of T helper (T_H) cells have been differentiated on the basis of cytokine secretion: the T_H1 subset secretes IL-2 and IFNγ; T_H2 subset cells produce IL-4, IL-5, IL-6 and IL-10. T_H1 cells are important in cytotoxic T cell responses, including protection against intracellular organisms and type IV hypersensitivity reactions. T_H2 cells promote antibody production by stimulating B cells.

Type II (cell-bound) hypersensitivity reactions occur when circulating

IgG or IgM antibodies bind to specific cell surface antigens. Once bound, these immunoglobulins can activate complement and thereby cause tissue damage. Examples include myasthenia gravis, Goodpasture's disease and autoimmune haemolytic anaemia. Grave's disease is classified as a **type V hypersensitivity** response since the long-acting thyroid stimulator IgG autoantibodies are stimulatory.

4.21 (a) F (b) F (c) F (d) T (e) F

Interferons are involved in limiting the spread of viral infections. All interferons have anti-viral activity but this is weaker in IFNγ than IFNα or IFNβ. IFNα and IFNβ are produced by cells which have become infected with virus: IFNα by leukocytes and IFNβ by fibroblasts. IFNγ is produced by activated T lymphocytes and natural killer (NK) cells. IFNγ activates macrophages, T_C cells, promotes differentiation of B cells (but inhibits proliferation), increases NK cell activity and increases all antigen presenting cell function by enhancing MHC class I and II antigen expression. IFNα and IFNβ have some anti-tumour activity, being capable of inhibiting cell growth in renal cell carcinoma and hairy cell leukaemia. IFNα is used in the treatment of hepatitis C infection. Excess IFNγ may be important in the development of autoimmune disease.

4.22 (a) T (b) T (c) T (d) T (e) T

The interleukins are a group of proteins, numbered IL-1 to IL-17, produced mainly by lymphocytes.

IL-1 is made predominantly by macrophages. It plays an important role in induction of the inflammatory response by stimulating T and B cell proliferation, and production of IL-2, γIFN and prostaglandins by T helper cells. IL-1 is an endogenous pyrogen, acting in the hypothalamus to cause fever, and stimulates bone resorption by osteoclasts.

IL-2 is produced by T cells (mainly CD4+). It is the most potent activator and growth factor of T cells, but also promotes growth and differentiation of B cells and activates macrophages.

IL-3 is produced by T cells and stimulates growth of all haemopoietic stem cells.

IL-4 is synthesized by T cells and is a stimulator of T_H2 cell differentiation and of B cell growth and differentiation. It is particularly potent in stimulating the production of IgE and IgG_1. It suppresses production of IL-1 and TNFα, and induces macrophage MHC class II expression. IL-10 is also an inhibitory interleukin.

IL-5 is an eosinophil growth and activation factor.

IL-6 stimulates B cell differentiation, acute phase protein synthesis, and is important in stimulating abnormal plasma cell clones in multiple myeloma.

4.23 (a) T (b) F (c) T (d) F (e) F
Physiological changes in response to infection include general malaise, anorexia, fever, polyarthralgia, increased metabolic rate and increased cardiac output. Biochemical changes include a fall in serum iron and zinc and increased hepatic production of acute phase proteins (C-reactive protein (readily monitored), orosomucoid and α_1-glycoprotein). Most of these changes occur in response to cytokines, predominantly IL-1, IL-6 and TNF. In Gram-negative infections endotoxin is a potent stimulator of TNF release, as are the cell walls of Gram-positive organisms. The response to viral infections is much less marked. Although there is evidence that the acute phase response has some protective function against infection, excess cytokine production can cause vascular damage and contributes to the clinical features of septicaemic shock. This syndrome can be prevented experimentally with the use of anti-TNF antibodies. C3b has a very short half-life.

4.24 (a) T (b) T (c) T (d) T (e) T
The genes for the ABO blood group system are on the long arm of chromosome 9. ABO blood types are determined by testing the erythrocytes with anti-A and anti-B antibodies, and by testing the serum against known A, B and O cells. Antibodies to blood group antigens other than one's own occur naturally (i.e. without prior exposure to antigen), and are IgM class immunoglobulins. Percentages of phenotypes vary between different populations and ethnic groups e.g. South American Indians all have blood group O (Table 4.2). Gastric carcinoma and pernicious anaemia are more common in individuals of blood group A. Peptic ulceration is more common in group O non-secretors. The rhesus (Rh) protein blood group locus is on chromosome 1. Rhesus antigen D is the most immunogenic in this grouping system. Anti-D antibody can induce severe transfusion reactions and haemolytic disease of the newborn. Monoclonal cold-agglutinating

Table 4.2 The ABO blood group system

Blood group	Phenotype frequency (%) in Caucasians	Antigen on cell surface	Agglutinin in plasma
A	42	A	Anti-B
B	8	B	Anti-A
AB	3	A+B	None
O	47	O	Anti-A, Anti-B

antibodies (anti-I) to the I antigen of the red cell membrane may develop after infection with *Mycoplasma pneumoniae*.

4.25 (a) T (b) T (c) T (d) F (e) T

Renal transplantation

In determining graft survival, matching for MHC class II antigens is more important than matching for class I antigens. ABO compatibility is also essential. Patients who have received multiple blood transfusions before operation have a lower incidence of graft failure. Hyperacute graft rejection occurs within minutes or hours, and is because of an antibody response against donor MHC class I antigens. Acute rejection occurs up to 3 months after transplantation and is because of a type IV hypersensitivity-type response. Chronic rejection is seen months or years after successful transplantation.

Bone marrow transplantation

The best outcome is when a complete match of chromosome 6 (the MHC) is made, e.g. from identical twin or sibling (there is a one in four chance of two siblings having the same HLA haplotype). Graft *versus* host disease (GVHD) occurs 7–14 days after transplantation. T cell depletion of donor marrow before transplantation reduces the incidence of GVHD, but increases the incidence of graft failure and relapse of the leukaemia.

Cardiac and liver transplantation

HLA matching is not necessary. Early diagnosis of rejection of the transplanted heart is essential. In early rejection endomyocardial biopsies typically show greatly increased MHC class I expression by myocytes.

Cyclosporin A blocks production of IL-2 by T_H (CD4+) cells. As a result the T_H cell response and natural killer cell activity is reduced leading to decreased incidence of graft rejection and GVHD.

FURTHER READING

Chapel, H. and Heaney, M. (1993) *Essentials of Clinical Immunology*, 3rd edn, Blackwell Scientific Publications, Oxford.

Hoffbrand, A.V. and Pettit, J.E. (1993) *Essential Haematology*, 3rd edn, Blackwell Scientific Publications, Oxford.

Roitt, I. Brostoff, J. and Male, D. (1996) *Immunology*, 4th edn, Mosby, London.

Russell, N.J., Powell, G., Jones, G., Winterburn, P.J. and Basford, J.M. (1982) *Blood Biochemistry*, Croom Helm, London.

5 Infectious diseases and HIV

QUESTIONS

5.1 The following are DNA viruses:
(a) herpes zoster virus.
(b) togaviruses.
(c) adenoviruses.
(d) rhabdoviruses.
(e) human immunodeficiency virus-1 (HIV-1).

5.2 The following statements regarding Lancefield group A streptococci are true:
(a) they are motile, spore-forming organisms.
(b) they are alpha-haemolytic.
(c) most pathogenic strains in humans are *Streptococcus pyogenes*.
(d) infection can result in non-infectious sequelae.
(e) they produce hyaluronidase as an extracellular product.

5.3 A girl of 16 years, previously well, develops pneumonia. The most likely causative organisms include:
(a) *Haemophilus influenzae*.
(b) *Pseudomonas aeruginosa*.
(c) *Streptococcus pneumoniae*.
(d) *Mycoplasma pneumoniae*.
(e) *Staphylococcus aureus*.

5.4 The following are insect-borne diseases:
(a) Dengue fever.
(b) filariasis.
(c) onchocerciasis.
(d) lymphogranuloma venereum.
(e) schistosomiasis.

5.5 The following are tick-borne diseases:
(a) trypanosomiasis.
(b) Lyme disease.
(c) Rocky Mountain spotted fever.
(d) fièvre boutonneuse.
(e) Dengue fever.

5.6 Minor criteria for the diagnosis of rheumatic fever include:
(a) P–R interval of 0.3 seconds.
(b) erythema chronicum migrans.
(c) chorea.
(d) positive streptococcal throat swab.
(e) polyarthritis.

5.7 The following are killed vaccines:
(a) pertussis.
(b) yellow fever.
(c) rubella.
(d) polio (Sabin).
(e) cholera.

5.8 The following infections occurring in pregnancy may result in foetal abnormalities:
(a) influenza A.
(b) rubella.
(c) cytomegalovirus.
(d) toxoplasmosis.
(e) hepatitis A.

5.9 Concerning acute hepatitis A virus infection:
(a) transmission is via the faeco-oral route.
(b) incubation period is 6 weeks to 3 months.
(c) jaundiced patients are highly infectious.
(d) diagnosis is confirmed by an acute rise in specific immunoglobulin G.
(e) chronic liver disease is a common sequel.

5.10 Regarding polio virus infection:
(a) transmission is primarily by respiratory droplet inhalation.
(b) 10% of those infected with the virus develop paralytic disease.
(c) tonsillectomy increases the incidence of bulbar disease.
(d) the majority of outbreaks are due to the type 2 strain.
(e) Salk inactivated polio vaccine is routinely used in the UK.

5.11 The following serum markers for hepatitis B virus would indicate that a patient is highly infectious:
(a) HBsAg-positive, HBeAg-positive.
(b) HBsAg-positive, anti-HBe-positive.
(c) Anti-HBc immunoglobulin M-positive.
(d) Anti-Hbc-positive, anti-HBe-positive.
(e) Anti-HBs-positive, anti-HBc-positive.

5.12 ***Vibrio cholerae***

(a) is a Gram-positive bacillus.
(b) invades the small intestine causing ulceration.
(c) toxin activates adenylate cyclase.
(d) causes profuse bloody diarrhoea.
(e) infection may cause a metabolic acidosis.

5.13 Hepatitis C:

(a) is a flavivirus.
(b) accounts for 90% of cases of non-A non-B hepatitis.
(c) is usually transmitted by sexual contact.
(d) infection may be associated with a low plasma C3 complement component.
(e) infection may be treated with interferon gamma.

5.14 Hepatitis E virus (HEV) infection:

(a) is caused by a flavivirus.
(b) is usually acquired in conjunction with hepatitis B.
(c) is associated with a long-term risk of chronic active hepatitis.
(d) during the third trimester of pregnancy is associated with a maternal mortality rate of approximately 30%.
(e) may be effectively treated with intravenous gammaglobulin.

5.15 The following statements regarding *Listeria monocytogenes* are true:

(a) the organism is a Gram-positive bacillus.
(b) *Listeria* can grow at –4°C.
(c) complement is the primary mode of host defence.
(d) serological tests are unhelpful in diagnosing infection.
(e) there is an increased risk of infection during the third trimester of pregnancy.

5.16 ***Escherichia coli* O157:H7**

(a) is a Gram-negative bacillus.
(b) typically causes travellers' diarrhoea.
(c) is a normal constituent of the bowel flora.
(d) is a common cause of haemolytic uraemic syndrome in children.
(e) infected patients are at risk of developing thrombotic thrombocytopenic purpura (TTP).

5.17 The following features are typical of acute brucellosis:
(a) leukopenia.
(b) normal erythrocyte sedimentation rate (ESR).
(c) hepatic granulomata on liver biopsy.
(d) agglutinins to *Proteus* OX-19.
(e) positive *Brucella* skin test.

5.18 Human immunodeficiency virus-1 (HIV-1):
(a) is a rhabdovirus.
(b) does not infect macrophages.
(c) *gag* and *env* genes code for structural proteins.
(d) p24 polypeptide is the chief component of the inner nucleocapsid.
(e) binds specifically to the CD8 membrane antigen on T helper cells.

5.19 The following statements are true:
(a) a fall in the CD8:CD4 ratio indicates HIV disease progression.
(b) there is a low level of viral replication in lymphoid tissue during the asymptomatic phase of HIV disease.
(c) low serum β_2-microglobulin levels are associated with increased risk of progression to AIDS.
(d) elevated levels of neopterin have been correlated to advancing clinical HIV disease.
(e) disease progression is slower in hereozygotes for the *CCR*-5 gene.

5.20 During HIV seroconversion illness:
(a) most patients are HIV-1 antibody-positive.
(b) immunoglobulin levels are low.
(c) the number of CD8 cells rises acutely.
(d) the CD4 cell count usually falls acutely.
(e) the level of HIV p24 antigen in the plasma will be low.

5.21 The following statements regarding the complications of HIV disease are true:
(a) lymphoma is commonly of the T cell type.
(b) Kaposi's sarcoma is caused by infection with human herpes virus type 8.
(c) *Cryptosporidium* is a well recognized cause of meningitis.
(d) cytomegalovirus (CMV) retinitis should be treated with high-dose intravenous acyclovir.
(e) molluscum contagiosum is caused by a pox virus.

5.22 *Pneumocystis carinii:*
(a) is an obligate intracellular parasite.
(b) infection is diagnosed by a fourfold rise in the antibody titre.
(c) infection in HIV is confined to the lungs.
(d) pneumonia (PCP) usually presents with lobar consolidation on the chest radiograph.
(e) prophylaxis should be started in HIV-positive patients with CD4 T cell counts of 200 cells/mm^3 or under.

5.23 Regarding central nervous system (CNS) disease in patients with AIDS:
(a) cerebral toxoplasmosis is more common in individuals with circulating antibodies to *Toxoplasma gondii.*
(b) progressive multifocal leukoencephalopathy is caused by a papilloma virus.
(c) neurons are unaffected in progressive multifocal leukoencephalopathy.
(d) HIV can be isolated from brain tissue in AIDS encephalopathy.
(e) primary CNS lymphoma is frequently associated with Epstein Barr virus (EBV) infection.

5.24 Zidovudine:
(a) is an analogue of thymidine.
(b) excretion is reduced by probenecid.
(c) treatment is typically associated with a rise in the mean corpuscular volume (MCV).
(d) causes dose-dependent bone marrow suppression.
(e) is contraindicated in pregnancy.

5.25 Regarding current anti-retroviral therapy:
(a) nucleoside analogues inhibit viral integrase.
(b) protease inhibitors prevent maturation of virions.
(c) non-nucleoside reverse transcriptase inhibitors bind directly to the HIV-1 reverse transcriptase enzyme.
(d) protease inhibitors induce cytochrome P450 enzymes.
(e) protease inhibitors are contraindicated in patients taking nucleoside analogues.

ANSWERS

5.1 (a) T (b) F (c) T (d) F (e) F

DNA viruses (mainly dsDNA)

Poxviruses	Variola, molluscum contagiosum

Herpes viruses	Herpes simplex, varicella zoster, Epstein Barr virus, cytomegalovirus
Adenoviruses	Adenovirus
Papovaviruses (ss)	Papilloma, polyoma
Parvoviruses	Human parvovirus B19
Hepnaviruses	Hepatitis B

RNA viruses (mainly ssRNA)

Orthomyxoviruses	Influenza
Paramyxoviruses	Parainfluenza, respiratory syncitial virus (RSV), measles, mumps
Rhabdoviruses	Rabies
Picornaviruses	Enteroviruses, poliovirus, Coxsackie, echovirus, hepatitis A, hepatitis E
Togaviruses	Rubella, alphaviruses
Flaviviruses	Hepatitis C, Yellow fever, Dengue fever
Reoviruses (ds)	Rotavirus
Arenaviruses	Lymphocytic choriomeningitis, Lassa fever
Retroviruses	HIV-1 and -2
Filoviruses	Marburg virus, Ebola virus

ss, Single stranded; ds, double stranded.

5.2 (a) F (b) F (c) T (d) T (e) T

Group A streptococci are non-spore-forming, β-haemolytic and most pathogenic strains in humans are *S. pyogenes*. The organism may cause tonsillitis, pharyngitis, peritonsillar abscess, scarlet fever, otitis media, mastoiditis, puerperal sepsis, cellulitis and impetigo. Infection may result in a number on non-infective sequelae, including rheumatic fever, erythema nodosum and glomerulonephritis. Numerous bacterial toxins are responsible for the pathogenicity of the organism; these include hyaluronidase, DNAases, haemolysins O and S, and erythrogenic toxins. These enzymes may be used for laboratory diagnosis.

5.3 (a) F (b) F (c) T (d) T (e) F

Mycoplasma and *Streptococcus pneumoniae* are the most likely causes of pneumonia in this patient. *Haemophilus influenzae* usually causes pneumonia secondary to pre-existing airways disease. *Pseudomonas aeruginosa* usually occurs in hospitalized, debilitated, immunosuppressed or ventilated patients, and also in cystic fibrosis. *Staphylococcus aureus* may follow infection with influenza, but is a frequent complication in patients with cystic fibrosis.

5.4 (a) T (b) T (c) T (d) F (e) F

Schistosomiasis is spread to man by cercariae penetrating skin, usually of the foot; a water snail is the intermediate vector. Lymphogranuloma venereum, caused by *Chlamydia trachomatis*, is sexually transmitted. Other insect-borne diseases are given in Table 5.1.

Table 5.1 Insect-borne diseases

Insect	Disease	Organism	Treatment
Tsetse fly (*Glossina* sp.)	African trypanosomiasis	*Trypanosoma brucei gambiense* and *rhodesiense*	Suramin, melarsoprol
Triatomine (Reduviid bugs)	American trypanosomiasis (Chagas disease)	*T. cruzi*	Nifurtinox, Benzidazole
Aedes mosquito	Yellow fever, Dengue fever		
Blackflies (*Simulium* sp.)	Onchocerciasis	*Onchocerca volvulus*	Ivermectin, suramin
Sandfly	Visceral leishmaniasis (kala-azar)	*Leishmania donovani*	Sodium stibogluconate
Deerfly (*Chrysops silacea*)	Loiasis	*Loa loa*	Diethylcarbamazine
Culex, Anopheles, and *Aedes* mosquitoes	Bancroftian filariasis	*Wuchereria bancrofti*	Diethylcarbamazine
Anopheles and *Mansonia* mosquitoes	Filariasis	*Brugia malayi* and *B. timori*	Diethylcarbamazine
Anopheles mosquitoes	Malaria	*Plasmodium flaciparum, vivax* and *ovale*	Varies according to type

5.5 (a) F (b) T (c) T (d) T (e) F

Disease	**Organism**
Rocky Mountain spotted fever	*Rickettsia rickettsii*
Fièvre boutonneuse	*Rickettsia conorii*
Q fever	*Coxiella burnetti*
Tularaemia	*Francisella tularensis*

Lyme disease	*Borrelia burgdorferi*
Tick-borne encephalitis	Flavivirus
Louping ill	Flavivirus
Human babesiosis	*Babesia* sp.
Tick paralysis	
Tick-borne haemorrhagic fevers:	
Kyasanur forest disease (India)	
Omsk haemorrhagic fever (USSR)	
Crimea-Congo haemorrhagic fever (Africa, E. Europe, Middle East, Asia)	

Trypanosomiasis and Dengue fever are insect-borne diseases (see previous question).

5.6 (a) T (b) F (c) F (d) F (e) F
The criteria for the diagnosis of rheumatic fever are shown in Table 5.2.

Table 5.2 American Heart Association – Jones criteria, 1992 update

Major criteria	Minor criteria	Supporting evidence of antecedent streptococcal infection
Carditis	Arthralgia	Positive throat culture or rapid streptococcal antigen test
Polyarthritis	Fever	
Chorea	Elevated ESR	
Erythema marginatum	Elevated CRP	
Subcutaneous nodules	Prolonged P–R interval	Elevated or rising streptococcal antigen titre

ESR, erythrocyte sedimentation rate.
CRP, C-reactive protein.

If supported by evidence of preceding group A streptococcal infection, the presence of two major manifestations or of one major and two minor manifestations indicates a high probability of acute rheumatic fever.

Erythema chronicum migrans is the acute rash associated with Lyme disease.

5.7 (a) T (b) F (c) F (d) F (e) T
Killed vaccines include diphtheria/tetanus/pertussis (DTP), polio (Salk), typhoid, cholera and hepatitis B.

Live vaccines include measles/mumps/rubella (MMR), yellow fever and polio (Sabin). Live vaccines are generally contraindicated in pregnant women and in immunosuppressed patients. Patients with HIV infection should not be given Bacille-Calmette-Guérin (BCG) or yellow fever vaccines, but can receive MMR and polio live vaccines.

Recommended schedule for childhood immunization in the UK (1997)

Diphtheria/Tetanus/Pertussis (DTP) and Polio

1st dose	2 months
2nd dose	3 months
3rd dose	4 months
DT and polio booster	3–5 years (primary school entry)
DT and polio booster	15–18 years (on leaving school)

Measles/Mumps/Rubella (MMR)

1st dose	12–18 months
2nd dose	3–5 years (primary school entry)

Rubella immunization should be given to 10–14-year-old girls who have not had MMR.

Haemophilus influenzae type b (Hib)

1st dose	2 months
2nd dose	3 months
3rd dose	4 months

Hib vaccine can be given as a single dose to children aged 13 months to 2 years who have not been immunized previously. The vaccine is not recommended in children over 4 years of age.

Bacille-Calmette-Guérin (BCG)

Single dose	10–14 years

This is given if a tuberculin test is negative. It is no longer given routinely in many areas.

5.8 (a) F (b) T (c) T (d) T (e) F

A number of maternal infections adversely affect the foetus *in utero*. These are known collectively as the TORCH infections: **T**oxoplasmosis, **O**ther (syphilis, HIV-1), **R**ubella, **C**ytomegalovirus (CMV) and **H**erpes. Toxoplasmosis affects the foetus in 40% of maternal infections. Infants may have hydrocephalus or microcephaly, associated with hepatomegaly, jaundice and thrombocytopenia. Rubella may result in congenital defects if contracted during the first 16 weeks of pregnancy. The defects comprise a triad of cataracts, nerve deafness and cardiac abnormalities, including patent ductus arteriosus, ventricular septal defect and tetralogy of Fallot. The infants may also have hepatosplenomegaly, jaundice, anaemia, thrombocytopenia and haemolytic anaemia. The brain is usually affected, causing microcephaly, and surviving infants are usually mentally retarded. CMV infection is the most common cause of congenital viral infection, affecting approximately 1–2% of live births. The spectrum of disease is wide – most babies are unaffected, but babies born to non-immune mothers may develop cytomegalic inclusion disease, characterized by jaundice, hepatosplenomegaly, a petechial rash and multiorgan involvement. Neurological effects can range from mild neurological changes to severe microcephaly.

5.9 (a) T (b) F (c) F (d) F (e) F
Hepatitis A virus is an RNA virus (picornavirus). Transmission is by faeco-oral route – many cases are mild with only gastrointestinal upset and no jaundice. Infection typically affects children, and large outbreaks may occur in institutions. The incubation time is 2–6 weeks (6 weeks to 6 months for hepatitis B). The virus is excreted for 2 weeks before the onset of the jaundice, but for only a few days after the onset of symptoms. Antibody to hepatitis A virus appears at the time of onset of jaundice and diagnosis is made by a rise in specific immunoglobulin M. Virus can also be detected in stool. Chronic infection does not occur and fulminant hepatitis is rare. The overall mortality rate is very low (0.1–0.2%).

5.10 (a) F (b) F (c) T (d) F (e) F
Polio-virus type 1 is responsible for most outbreaks of paralytic polio, whilst type 2 is the strongest immunogen. The faeco-oral route is the primary mode of transmission, and the organism is stable in food, milk and water. Of those infected, 90–95% are asymptomatic as the virus is contained in the regional lymph nodes, 4–8% experience a mild flu-like illness, and 1–2% a major aseptic meningitis, of whom a small proportion will go on and develop classical paralytic polio. The virus affects the anterior horn cells of the spinal cord, cranial nuclei of the brainstem, and cells of the motor cortex. Tonsillectomy increases the risk of bulbar polio. The virus may be cultured from stools up to 5 weeks after onset of the illness. The diagnosis is confirmed by a fourfold rise in antibody titre between acute and convalescent sera. Cerebrospinal fluid shows high protein, normal glucose and initially polymorphs but later a lymphocytosis. Live oral polio vaccine (Sabin)

is used in the UK: the virus multiplies in the gut, stimulating local production of immunoglobulin A in addition to serum anti-bodies. Inactivated vaccine (Salk) is used in the USA.

5.11 (a) T (b) F (c) T (d) F (e) F

A large excess of HBsAg is produced in the liver during viral replication and is detectable in the patient's serum 6 weeks to 3 months after acute infection, and 2–8 weeks before any abnormality develops in liver function tests. Its presence suggests either current infection, chronic infection or carrier state. As the acute illness progresses, increasing amounts of HBeAg and viral DNA polymerase become detectable in the blood. Presence of HBeAg is associated with more severe infection, and blood is highly infectious. HBcAg is rarely detected in serum and is largely confined to the infected hepatocyte.

Anti-HBc IgM is the first antibody to appear, and persists for 1–2 weeks before anti-HBc IgG appears. Presence of anti-HBc IgM indicates acute infection and on-going viral replication. Anti-HBe appears in the first 1–3 weeks, followed by loss of HBeAg, therefore indicating decreased infectivity. Six weeks to six months after the acute illness anti-HBs appears, followed by the disappearance of HBsAg, indicating immunity.

This sequence of antigen appearance, antibody response and antigen clearance can stop at any stage. Patients who fail to develop anti-HBe antibodies are potentially infectious, even if HBeAg clears spontaneously. Patients who are HBsAg-positive pose a lower, though significant, risk of infection. If antigens remain detectable after 6 months (5–10%) the patient is considered to be a chronic carrier of hepatitis B: those with persistent HBe antigenaemia, or those who fail to develop HBe antibody, are at risk of developing chronic active or chronic persistent hepatitis, cirrhosis and ultimately hepatocellular carcinoma.

5.12 (a) F (b) F (c) T (d) F (e) T

Cholera is mediated by a toxin produced by the O1 and O139 serotypes of *Vibrio cholerae*, a comma-shaped, motile, flagellate, Gram-negative bacillus. The O1 serotype exists in two biotypes, classical and El Tor. Cholera is an acute diarrhoeal illness which can result in rapid progressive dehydration and death within hours. Once established in the gut, vibrios produce a potent protein exotoxin, cholera toxin, consisting of two sub-units A and B. The B sub-unit binds to GM1 ganglioside, a glycolipid receptor located on the surface of jejunal epithelial cells. The A sub-unit activates the intracellular enzyme adenylate cyclase by activating a G protein in intestinal epithelial cells, resulting in accumulation of high levels of intracellular cyclic

AMP (cAMP). This elevation in cAMP inhibits sodium reabsorption and activates chloride excretion in villus cells leading to the secretion of massive amounts of isotonic fluid into the intestine. The diarrhoea is watery, non-bloody and frequently described as 'rice-water' stools. Fluid replacement is the mainstay of treatment. Antibiotics are not necessary to clear the infection, though will reduce the duration of the illness, the amount of fluid loss and reduce infectivity. Single-dose tetracycline or trimethoprim-sulphamethoxazole are suitable.

5.13 (a) T (b) T (c) F (d) T (e) F

Hepatitis C is a positive-stranded RNA virus of the family Flaviviridae. Most patients are asymptomatic, though some describe fatigue. There is seldom a history of an acute hepatitis or jaundice. The virus is usually transmitted parenterally, e.g. intravenous drug use, blood transfusion, blood products or needlestick injury. The incubation period is 7 weeks. Sexual transmission and vertical transmission have been described, but are unusual ($< 5\%$ of cases). The diagnosis relies on molecular biological techniques such as polymerase chain reaction to detect viral RNA, or immunoassays for hepatitis C antibodies. The treatment for hepatitis C infection is interferon-alpha, given as a subcutaneous injection. About 80% of patients develop normal serum aspartate transaminase levels while undergoing treatment, but a sustained response is seen in only 25%. Patients infected with virus type 1 are more likely to be resistant to interferon than those with types 2 or 3. Adjunctive treatment with the nucleoside analogue ribavirin may help to reduce relapse rates. Hepatitis C is the most common cause of essential mixed cryoglobulinaemia (IgG and IgM) typically presenting with a vasculitic skin rash. Raynaud's phenomenon and peripheral neuropathy, with a positive rheumatoid factor and low serum levels of the C3 complement component. Chronic hepatitis C infection may progress to cirrhosis (10–20%) and hepatocellular carcinoma (1–5%), usually over a period of 20 or more years.

5.14 (a) F (b) F (c) F (d) T (e) F

HEV is a single-stranded RNA picornavirus. It resembles hepatitis A in its enteric mode of spread, and the clinical picture is of an acute self-limiting illness which does not cause chronic infection. Cases usually occur after contamination of water supplies, which frequently causes large outbreaks. There is also a significant risk of vertical transmission. The incubation period is 5–6 weeks. HEV mainly affects young adults and usually has a low mortality rate (2%). However, this rises to 20–40% if HEV infection occurs during pregnancy (particularly in the third trimester); deaths are due to fulminant hepatitis. HEV is secreted in stool during the late incubation period and diagnosis is based on finding virions on electron microscopy. Treatment is supportive; gammaglobulin is ineffective. No vaccine exists at present. Hepatitis D (the delta agent) is a defective RNA virus which only exists in the presence of hepatitis B, and is acquired by the same route.

5.15 (a) T (b) F (c) F (d) T (e) T

Listeria monocytogenes is a Gram-positive bacillus. *Listeria* grow well at temperatures of 1–45°C: cases of listeriosis are usually food-borne as the organism is able to withstand refrigeration, and is a common contaminant in soft cheeses and unpasteurized milk. The organism is an intracellular pathogen and therefore has a predilection for individuals with impaired cell-mediated immunity. Most cases of listeriosis occur in the elderly, in pregnancy and in immunocompromised patients. The risk of acquiring the infection in pregnancy is 17 times that of the general population. Meningitis or meningioencephalitis is the most common mode of presentation. Cerebrospinal fluid usually shows a neutrophilia (or a monocytosis), high protein and normal glucose. Diagnosis is by culture – the organism grows within 36 h on routine culture media. Serological tests are unhelpful in diagnosis as the organism is ubiquitous and antibodies may not rise following infection. Ampicillin or penicillin is the treatment of choice.

5.16 (a) T (b) F (c) F (d) T (e) T

E. coli is a Gram-negative enteric bacillus, classified as enterotoxigenic (causing travellers' diarrhoea), enteropathic, enteroinvasive and enterohaemorrhagic. All enterohaemorrhagic strains belong to the serotype O157:H7, designated by the somatic (O) and flagellar (H) antigens, and cause haemorrhagic colitis. The organism adheres to the gut mucosa and produces vero-cytotoxin (also termed Shiga-like toxin), which acts both locally on the gut and systematically. Most outbreaks have been due to the consumption of infected, undercooked beef. The incubation period is 3–4 days. Clinically, patients present with cramping abdominal pain and bloody diarrhoea. Patients may be apyrexial or have a low-grade fever. Haemolytic uraemic syndrome (HUS) develops in about 6% of cases, usually in children or the elderly. *E. coli* O157:H7 is the commonest cause of HUS in children in the UK and North America, and has a mortality rate of 2–10%. TTP occurs more frequently in adults and has similar clinical features to HUS, though the renal damage is less severe and neurological signs are prominent. The mortality rate from *E. coli* O157:H7 infection is 3–5%; 5% of surviving patients have permanent renal or neurological impairment.

5.17 (a) T (b) T (c) T (d) F (e) F

Brucella are small, non-motile, non-encapsulated Gram-negative coccobacilli. Human infection usually follows occupational exposure to an infected animal, or from ingestion of infected animal products (particularly unpasteurized milk). Four species of *Brucella* cause disease in man: *B. melitensis* (sheep and goats) is the most pathogenic, followed by *B. abortus* (cattle), *B. suis* (pigs) and *B. canis* (dogs). Granulomata form in response to Brucella infection, usually in the reticuloendothelial system (liver, spleen and bone marrow). The symptoms of acute brucellosis are non-specific, and are often without physical signs. Routine laboratory tests may be unhelpful: the white cell count is usually normal or low; the ESR may be normal. Diagnosis relies mainly on serological tests: a fourfold rise in antibodies to *Brucella* lipopolysaccharide antigens indicates recent exposure. The *Brucella* skin test is a measure of previous infection and can confuse the results of agglutination assays by causing a rise in antibody levels. Agglutinins to *Proteus* OX-19 develop in rickettsial diseases (particularly Rocky Mountain spotted fever and murine typhus) and form the basis of the Weil–Felix reaction.

5.18 (a) F (b) F (c) T (d) T (e) F

HIV-1 is a retrovirus of the subgroup lentivirus. The icosahedral outer capsid bears 72 spikes, formed by the two major viral envelope proteins gp120 and gp41. Human T helper (CD4+) lymphocytes are specifically infected by HIV because the CD4 membrane antigen is the principal high-affinity receptor for the gp120 envelope protein. The coffin-shaped inner capsid is bound by the nucleocapsid protein, p24, and contains other proteins (p7, p9 and p17), two copies of viral ssRNA and the enzymes reverse transcriptase, polymerase and integrase, which are essential for viral replication. Other cells infected by HIV include glial cells, gut epithelium and bone marrow progenitors. Infection of these may contribute, respectively, to the dementia, wasting syndrome and haematological abnormalities seen in HIV. HIV-1 also infects monocytes and macrophages, which become a major reservoir for the virus, although it has a much less pronounced cytopathic effect on these cells.

The HIV-1 *gag* gene encodes the core nucleocapsid polypeptides (p24, p7, p9 and p17). The *env* gene encodes the exterior coat proteins (gp120 and gp41). The *pol* gene encodes the viral reverse transcriptase, polymerase and integrase enzymes. (HIV-1 also contains at least six other regulatory genes (*vif*, *vpu*, *vpr*, *tat*, *rev* and *nef*).

5.19 (a) F (b) F (c) F (d) T (e) T

The normal CD4 count in adults is in the range 600–1500 cells/mm^3. The absolute CD4 count is usually used for staging disease, though a fall in the CD4:CD8 ratio also reflects disease progression. β_2-Microglobulin is a protein present on the surface of all nucleated cells, as the light chain of class I MHC. Levels of β_2-microglobulin are increased during mononuclear cell activation or destruction. Neopterin is produced during GTP metabolism, primarily by monocytes and macrophages. Elevated levels of neopterin and β_2-microglobulin have been correlated to disease progression. Following primary infection with HIV, the patient enters a clinically latent period lasting approximately 5–10 years. Although there are low levels of HIV in the plasma, the rate of replication in lymphoid tissue is extremely high.

Although the CD4 receptor is the principal binding site of HIV-1, several other co-receptors are also required for infection. The most important of these are the receptors CCR-5 and fusin. Fusin is a G protein-coupled cell receptor for T cell tropic strains of HIV. CCR-5 is the second receptor for macrophage-tropic strains of HIV. Individuals with homozygous base-pair deletions in the *CCR*-5 gene are resistant to infection with HIV-1; heterozygotes appear to have slower disease progression.

5.20 (a) F (b) F (c) T (d) T (e) F

Between 2 and 4 weeks after infection with HIV, 50–60% of patients develop an acute illness associated with seroconversion. The clinical picture is variable, but the most common symptoms and signs include fever (97%), lymphadenopathy (66%), pharyngitis (73%), erythematous maculopapular rash (70%) and myalgia or arthralgia (58%). During the first 2 weeks of the illness there is a lymphopenia; CD4 levels may be as low as those in advanced HIV disease. This is followed by a lymphocytosis, primarily consisting of CD8 cells. Although IgM anti-HIV antibodies (to Gag and Env proteins) usually appear within 2 weeks of infection, IgG antibodies are not detectable for 2–4 weeks after infection. Of patients infected with HIV, 95% have seroconverted within 5.6 months. Assay for p24 antigen is very useful in establishing a diagnosis of primary HIV-1 infection. High levels of p24 antigen may be detectable within 24 h of onset of the illness, and is always detectable before Gag and Env antibodies appear. Immunoglobulin levels are usually normal until the later stages of AIDS.

5.21 (a) F (b) T (c) F (d) F (e) T

Lymphoma develops in 3% of patients with HIV during the course of their illness. Generally, it occurs later in the disease with CD4 cell counts of 200 cells/mm^3 or less. Non-Hodgkin's lymphoma (NHL), Hodgkin's disease (HD) and primary central nervous system lymphoma (PCNSL) are all recognized in associations with HIV. Most HIV-positive patients with lymphoma have high-grade B cell NHL. Herpes virus-8 gene sequences have recently been isolated from Kaposi's sarcoma (KS) lesions in patients with AIDS. The virus is probably sexually transmitted – this is supported by the observation that KS is rare in intravenous drug abusers and haemophiliacs with HIV. In HIV, 66% of KS lesions are around the nose and mouth. Meningitis caused by the fungus *Cryptococcus neoformans* is well described; *Cryptosporidium* causes a diarrhoeal illness. Infection with CMV occurs late in the disease (CD4 counts of 100 cells/mm^3 or less), and may present as retinitis, colitis, sclerosing cholangitis, pneumonitis or adrenalitis. CMV is treated with either intravenous ganciclovir or foscarnet.

5.22 (a) F (b) F (c) F (d) F (e) T

Pneumocystis carinii was originally classified as a protozoan, but is more closely related to yeasts. *Pneumocystis carinii* pneumonia (PCP) is the commonest manifestation of disease: 70–80% of patients with HIV develop at least one episode of PCP during the course of their disease. The mortality rate ranges from 10 to 50% for each episode, depending on severity. PCP is most commonly seen in patients with CD4 cell counts of 200 cells/mm^3 or less. Clinical presentation is with fever, dyspnoea and a non-productive cough. Auscultation of the chest may be normal. Chest radiographs are commonly normal, even with severe PCP, or may show a bilateral hilar interstitial infiltrate. PCP is complicated by pneumothorax in 2% of cases. The diagnosis is made by isolating trophozoites or cyst forms from either induced sputum, bronchoalveolar lavage, transbronchial biopsy or open lung biopsy. The treatment of choice for PCP is cotrimoxazole (Septrin), either orally or parenterally, depending on the severity of disease. Alternatives to cotrimoxazole include intravenous pentamidine, trimethoprim with dapsone, and clindamycin with primaquine. Corticosteroids have been shown to improve the prognosis in patients with $Pa_{O2} < 10$ kPa (70 mmHg). PCP prophylaxis should be started when the patient's CD4 count falls to 200 cells/mm^3. The first-line prophylactic agent is cotrimoxazole taken once daily. Long-term treatment invariably results in intolerance. Alternatives include aerosolized pentamidine or dapsone.

5.23 (a) T (b) F (c) F (d) T (e) T

Cerebral toxoplasmosis is the most common cause of focal CNS pathology in AIDS, causing disease in 15% of patients with AIDS. It is thought to be because of reactivation of dormant *Toxoplasma gondii*, as clinical disease is 10 times more common in patients with antibodies to the organism. Infection occurs in the later stages of HIV disease (CD4 count < 100 cells/mm^3). Cerebral toxoplasmosis appears as multiple ring-enhancing lesions on magnetic resonance imaging or contrast computed tomography, occasionally with mass effect and oedema. Definitive diagnosis is by brain biopsy, though treatment is usually initiated on the basis of clinical and radiographic findings. Treatment is with sulphadiazine and pyrimethamine (and folinic acid) and should be life-long as the relapse rate is 50% at 6 months.

The incidence of non-Hodgkin's lymphoma (NHL) in patients with AIDS appears to be increasing. Primary CNS lymphoma (PCNSL) typically occurs in late-stage disease (CD4 < 50 cells/mm^3). Untreated, PCNSL has a median survival of 1.5 months, increasing to only 5 months with radiotherapy and/or chemotherapy. EBV genomic proteins are almost invariably found in PCNSL, compared with 50% of AIDS-associated NHL.

Progressive multifocal leukoencephalopathy is the third major cause of focal CNS pathology in AIDS. It is an opportunistic disease caused by infection with a human papovavirus, named JC virus, the initials of the patient from whom the virus was first isolated. It occurs in late-stage AIDS (CD4 count < 200 cells/mm^3). Oligodendrocytes, the source of CNS myelin, are the main cells affected, leading to demyelination. Definitive diagnosis is on brain biopsy. No specific treatment has proven effective and the prognosis is extremely poor.

5.24 (a) T (b) T (c) T (d) T (e) F

Zidovudine (3′-azido-2′,3′-dideoxythymidine, AZT) is a nucleoside analogue. Zidovudine is triphosphorylated in infected and uninfected cells by thymidine kinase. Zidovudine triphosphate acts as a substrate for, and an inhibitor of, viral reverse transcriptase by acting as a DNA chain terminator. Bone marrow suppression is dose-dependent. AZT also has a high affinity for human mitochondrial DNA polymerase, which may contribute to the myopathy or myositis which is occasionally seen on treatment. Other side effects include insomnia and blue pigmentation of the nails. An elevated MCV is a common finding in patients taking AZT. Hepatic microsomal enzyme inducers and inhibitors may alter the metabolism of zidovudine. Probenecid reduces renal excretion of zidovudine metabolites and also decreases hepatic glucuronidation, thereby increasing its half-life.

HIV is transmitted from an infected mother to her foetus in approximately 30% of cases. Although transmission can occur across the placenta, it is thought that most vertical transmission occurs in the perinatal period. Zidovudine given to HIV-positive pregnant women (orally antepartum, and as an intravenous infusion during delivery) and their babies (orally to the neonate for 6 weeks) has reduced the rate of transmission to < 10%.

5.25 (a) F (b) T (c) T (d) F (e) F
Nucleoside analogues inhibit viral reverse transcriptase and terminate the developing DNA chain; protease inhibitors prevent maturation of virions; non-nucleoside reverse transcriptase inhibitors bind to HIV-1 reverse transcriptase. Protease inhibitors inhibit the cytochrome P450 enzyme pathway, thereby increasing plasma concentrations of other drugs metabolized by the same system, including diazepam, terfenadine and amiodarone. Ritonavir is the most potent inhibitor of cytochrome P450 enzymes. Recent studies have clearly shown that combination therapy with two or three anti-retroviral agents is far more effective in reducing viral load and preventing disease progression than monotherapy. The high error rate of reverse transcriptase means that monotherapy simply selects drug-resistant mutants. Combinations typically consist of two nucleoside analogues (one of which is usually AZT) and a protease inhibitor.

FURTHER READING

Boyce, T.F., Swerdlow, D.L. and Griffin, P.M. (1995) *Escherichia coli* O157:H7 and the haemolytic uraemic syndrome. *New Engl J Med,* **333**, 364–8.

Cohn, J.A. (1997) Recent advances: HIV-1 infection. *BMJ*, **314**, 487–91.

Deeks, S.G., Smith, M., Holodniy, M. and Kahn, J.O. (1997) HIV protease inhibitors: a review for clinicians. *JAMA* **277**, 145–53.

Denton, A.S., Brook, M.G. and Miller, R.F. (1996) AIDS-related lymphoma: an emerging epidemic. *Br J Hosp Med*, **55**, 282–8.

Dusheiko, G.M., Khakoo, S., Soni, P. and Greiller, L. (1996) A rational approach to the management of hepatitis C infection, *BMJ*, **312**, 357–64.

Gazzard, B.G., Moyle, G.I., Weber, J. *et al.* (1997) British HIV Association guidelines for antiretroviral treatment of HIV seropositive individuals, *Lancet*, **349** 1086–92.

Krawczynski, K. (1993) Hepatitis E. *Hepatology*, **17**, 932–41.

McNair, A.N.B., Tibbs, C.J. and Williams, R. (1995) Recent advances: hepatology. *BMJ*, **311**, 1351–5.

Sweeney, B.J., Miller, R.F. and Harrison, M.J.G. (1993) Progressive multifocal leucoencephalopathy, *Br J Hosp Med*, **50**, 187–191.
Major advances in the treatment of HIV-1 infection. *Drug and Therapeutics Bulletin*, 1997, **35**, 25–9.

6 Diabetes, endocrinology and metabolism

QUESTIONS

6.1 The following statements regarding non-insulin dependent diabetes mellitus (NIDDM) are correct:
(a) concordance for monozygotic twins is approximately 100%.
(b) 50% of cases are due to a mutation of the insulin gene.
(c) when it occurs in young people (maturity onset diabetes of the young [MODY]) it is autosomal dominant.
(d) it is associated with a mutation in mitochondrial DNA in some patients.
(e) the glucokinase gene has been implicated in its pathophysiology.

6.2 Insulin:
(a) is secreted by the alpha cells of the pancreas.
(b) is secreted with C peptide in equimolar amounts.
(c) secretion is stimulated by somatostatin.
(d) receptors have protein kinase activity.
(e) concentrations in plasma increase about 40 times after a 75 g oral glucose load.

6.3 Insulin:
(a) increases hepatic gluconeogenesis.
(b) increases muscle glycogen synthesis.
(c) is required for glucose uptake in all tissues.
(d) inhibits lipoprotein lipase.
(e) increases protein synthesis.

6.4 The following mechanisms mediate insulin action:
(a) cell membrane receptor interaction.
(b) adenylate cyclase activation.
(c) receptor tyrosine kinase activity.
(d) internalization of hormone-receptor complexes.
(e) hormone receptor DNA binding.

6.5 Insulin resistance:
(a) is associated with acanthosis nigricans.

(b) may be the result of defective synthesis and translocation of glucose transporters (GLUT).
(c) in obesity may improve with weight reduction.
(d) is associated with hypertension.
(e) is not a feature of Cushing's syndrome.

6.6 In diabetic ketoacidosis:
(a) there is complete insulin deficiency.
(b) there is excess hepatic glucose output.
(c) the circulating concentration of glucagon is reduced.
(d) ketones are mostly formed in adipose tissue.
(e) peripheral glucose extraction in muscle is reduced.

6.7 Diabetes mellitus may be a feature of:
(a) haemochromatosis.
(b) malnutrition.
(c) primary hyperaldosteronism.
(d) somatostatinoma.
(e) primary biliary cirrhosis.

6.8 The following statements regarding vitamin D are correct:
(a) vitamin D3 (cholecalciferol) is the natural form.
(b) 25-hydroxyvitamin D is converted to its active metabolite in the skin by ultraviolet light.
(c) it inhibits the effects of parathyroid hormone on bone.
(d) it has its primary effect on the intestine.
(e) formation of 1,25-dihydroxyvitamin D is reduced when plasma calcium is low.

6.9 Calcitonin:
(a) is a single chain polypeptide.
(b) is secreted by the parathyroid epithelial cells.
(c) secretion is increased by a fall in serum calcium concentration.
(d) inhibits bone resorption.
(e) is secreted in response to increased gastrin levels.

6.10 The following statements regarding phosphate metabolism are correct:
(a) the major route of excretion is via the intestine.
(b) it is reabsorbed in the kidney by the distal tubule.
(c) parathyroid hormone inhibits renal absorption of phosphate.
(d) absorption from the intestine is primarily by passive diffusion.
(e) over 60% of ingested phosphate is absorbed.

6.11 The following statements regarding circulating carrier proteins are true:

(a) 50% of circulating aldosterone is bound to albumin.
(b) transthyretin binds specifically to thyroxine.
(c) sex steroid-binding globulin has a low specificity for oestradiol.
(d) hormones bound to proteins have about 50% of the activity of the free hormone.
(e) α_2 macroglobulin is an important general carrier.

6.12 The following hormones are amino acid derivatives:

(a) noradrenaline.
(b) human chorionic gonadotrophin.
(c) aldosterone.
(d) melatonin.
(e) parathyroid hormone.

6.13 Membrane hormone receptors:

(a) are often glycoproteins.
(b) for insulin exhibit an intrinsic protein kinase activity.
(c) for glucagon have inisotol triphosphate (IP_3) as a second messenger.
(d) are coupled to adenylate cyclase by G proteins.
(e) can stimulate calcium ion transport into cells.

6.14 Growth hormone:

(a) is secreted in response to somatostatin released from the hypothalamus.
(b) is secreted in a steady continuous fashion.
(c) stimulates the production of somatomedins.
(d) secretion is stimulated by rapid eye movement (REM) sleep.
(e) increases hepatic gluconeogenesis.

6.15 Aldosterone secretion is:

(a) stimulated by potassium depletion.
(b) increased in response to hypovolaemia.
(c) increased following assumption of the upright posture.
(d) primary from cells in the zona fasciculata of the adrenal gland.
(e) decreased by the administration of adrenocorticotrophic hormone (ACTH).

6.16 Glucocorticoid hormones:

(a) are primarily carried in the blood by corticosteroid-binding globulin.
(b) bind to hormone receptors on cell membranes.
(c) increase liver gluconeogenesis.
(d) increase skeletal muscle synthesis.
(e) decrease adipose glucose uptake.

6.17 The following statements about lipoprotein metabolism are correct:

(a) dietary triglycerides are transported to the liver as very low density lipoproteins (VLDLs).
(b) cholesterol synthesis in the liver is controlled by 3-hydroxy-3-methylglutaryl coenzyme A (HMGCoA) reductase.
(c) high density lipoproteins are mostly made up of triglycerides.
(d) raised blood concentrations of lipoprotein a are associated with increased mortality from coronary heart disease.
(e) in people with heterozygous familial hypercholesterolaemia serum low density lipoprotein (LDL) concentrations are elevated from birth.

6.18 In the oxidation of glucose to carbon dioxide and water:

(a) the first stage of glycolysis consumes ATP.
(b) glycolysis yields about 3% of the free energy obtained.
(c) there is allosteric inhibition of citrate synthetase in the citric acid cycle by ATP.
(d) about 30% of adenosine triphosphate (ATP) is generated by oxidative phosphorylation.
(e) about 50 kcal/mol of energy is stored in each molecule of ATP.

6.19 During normal pregnancy:

(a) human chorionic gonadotrophin (hCG) is necessary for endometrial growth.
(b) maternal insulin secretion is increased in the first trimester.
(c) gonadotrophin releasing hormone (GnRH) secretion is increased.
(d) in the second trimester the placenta takes about 50% of cardiac output.
(e) there is increased activity of the renin/angiotensin system.

6.20 Vasopressin (antidiuretic hormone):
(a) is secreted by the anterior pituitary gland.
(b) is released when blood volume increases.
(c) release is inhibited by alcohol.
(d) is deficient in nephrogenic diabetes insipidus.
(e) increases extracellular fluid volume.

6.21 Leptin:
(a) is secreted by the anterior pituitary gland.
(b) inhibits synthesis and release of neuropeptide Y from the hypothalamus.
(c) concentrations in the plasma are related to body fat mass.
(d) concentrations in the plasma are related to the development of non-insulin dependent diabetes mellitus.
(e) suppresses fat ingestion.

6.22 Acute intermittent porphyria (AIP):
(a) is an autosomal recessive disorder.
(b) is more common in females.
(c) usually presents before puberty.
(d) is caused by abnormal function of δ-amino laevulinic acid (ALA) synthetase.
(e) results in the accumulation of porphobilinogen (PBG) in urine.

6.23 The thyroid stimulating hormone receptor (TSH-R):
(a) is the prime autoantigen in Graves' disease.
(b) uses cyclic adenosine monophosphate (c-AMP) as a second messenger.
(c) is blocked by antibodies in atrophic thyroiditis.
(d) antibodies are useful in predicting patients who will relapse after drug treatment for Graves' disease.
(e) is inhibited by thionamides such as carbimazole.

6.24 3,3′,5-tri-iodothyronine (T3):
(a) is synthesized from thyroglobulin.
(b) is very soluble in aqueous solutions.
(c) activates cell surface receptors.
(d) is only synthesized in the thyroid gland.
(e) is four times more active than 3,3′,5,5′-tetraiodothyronine (T4).

6.25 In the hypothalamus:
(a) neural connections are the main means of communication with the posterior part of the pituitary gland.

(b) somatostatin stimulates growth hormone secretion.
(c) oxytocin is synthesized in the supraoptic nuclei.
(d) only stimulating hormones are released to the anterior pituitary gland.
(e) dopamine inhibits prolactin release.

ANSWERS

6.1 (a) T (b) F (c) T (d) T (e) T

NIDDM affects 5–10% of the population in the western world. Problems do not usually arise until middle age and it is associated with obesity. Twin studies show almost 100% concordance, indicating a major hereditary component to this disorder. A number of mutations on chromosomes 6 and 19 have been linked with NIDDM, including the genes for adenosine deaminase and glucokinase. MODY is a variant condition in younger people and is autosomal dominant. In some patients with associated deafness a mutation in mitochondrial DNA has been described.

6.2 (a) F (b) T (c) F (d) T (e) F

Insulin is secreted from beta cells. (Alpha cells produce glucagon, delta cells make somatostatin and F cells produce pancreatic polypeptide.) Pro-insulin is synthesized first and then cleaved. An equal amount of the cleaved peptide segment 'C peptide' is released into the circulation. C peptide has no biological functions. Factors affecting secretion are listed below:

Stimulation	**Inhibition**
↑ blood glucose	Somatostatin
Amino acids	Catecholamines
Fatty acids	
Sulphonylureas	
Glucagon	
Acetylcholine	

The most important stimulation of insulin is blood glucose, and a 75 g glucose load results in about a 10-fold increase in insulin. Insulin binds to a membrane receptor with protein kinase activity and may phosphorylate regulatory proteins in target cells.

6.3 (a) F (b) T (c) F (d) F (e) T

Most tissues require insulin for glucose uptake, apart from brain and liver which are permeable to glucose in the absence of insulin.

The effects of insulin on metabolism in tissues are shown in Table 6.1.

Table 6.1 Effects of insulin on tissue metabolism

	Hepatic	Muscle	Adipose
Carbohydrate	↓ glucose release ↓ gluconeogeneis ↑ glycogen synthesis	↑ glucose uptake ↑ glycogen synthesis	↑ glucose uptake
Fat	↑ fatty acid synthesis ↑ storage of triglycerides		↑ fatty acid synthesis ↑ storage of triglycerides (via hormone sensitive lipase) ↑ uptake of lipoproteins (via lipoprotein lipase)
Protein	↑ amino acid uptake ↑ protein synthesis ↓ muscle degradation	↑ amino acid uptake ↑ protein synthesis (via ribosomal effect) ↓ muscle degradation	

6.4 (a) T (b) F (c) T (d) T (e) F

Insulin receptors are large glycoproteins with two alpha and two beta sub-units linked by disulphide bridges (Figure 6.1). The gene for insulin receptors is found on chromosome 19.

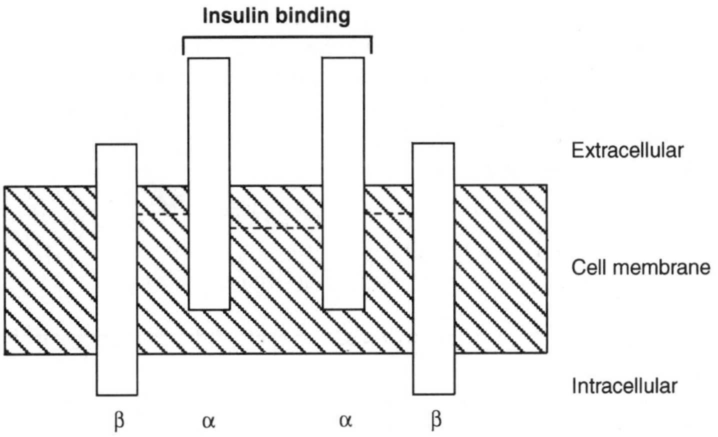

Figure 6.1 Structure of the insulin receptor.

After binding to the receptor the hormone–receptor complex is internalized and degraded with some receptor recycling.

Second messenger activity is via tyrosine kinase-mediated phosphorylation of tyrosine residues of cytosolic proteins. Autophosphorylation of receptor proteins occurs. Phosphorylation of proteins such as insulin receptor substrate-1 (IRS-1) may mediate intracellular actions of insulin. There is no hormone receptor DNA binding.

6.5 (a) T (b) T (c) T (d) T (e) F

Insulin resistance is associated with a number of rare conditions such as acanthosis nigricans and ataxia telangiectasia. It is an important factor in secondary diabetes because of increased catabolic hormones such as catecholamines, glucagon, cortisol and growth hormone. Glucose uptake into cells is mediated by facultative membrane glucose transporters (GLUTs). GLUT 1 provides basal glucose uptake, GLUT 2 is a feature of cells which release glucose as well as taking it up. GLUT 4 is found in muscle and adipose tissue and is the major transporter in insulin-sensitive tissues. There is evidence of an effect of insulin on GLUT 4 synthesis and translocation, and this may have a role in insulin resistance.

Insulin resistance is associated with non-insulin dependent diabetes mellitus, obesity, hypertriglyceridaemia and hypertension.

6.6 (a) F (b) T (c) F (d) F (e) T

Diabetic ketoacidosis (DKA) may be defined as a ketonaemia associated with a plasma bicarbonate of less than 15 mmol/l. It results from relative rather than complete insulinopenia. Insulin levels are around 10 U/l, which is approximately the level found after an overnight fast, but this is inappropriately low for a plasma glucose of 30–40 mmol/l. Catabolic hormones, catecholamines, glucagon, growth hormone and cortisol are elevated 3–10 times in DKA and have an important role in the development of the syndrome. The effects of insulinopenia and increased catabolic hormones are shown in Table 6.2.

6.7 (a) T (b) T (c) T (d) T (e) F

Secondary diabetes is a feature of the following disorders:

- pancreatic disease, e.g. cystic fibrosis, pancreatitis, carcinoma of the pancreas;
- haemochromatosis – due to iron deposition in islet cells;
- malnutrition, i.e. protein-deficient pancreatic diabetes and fibrocalculous pancreatic diabetes;
- drugs, e.g. thiazide diuretics, corticosteroids;

Table 6.2 Effects of insulinopenia and increased catabolic hormones

	Insulin	Catecholamines	Glucagon	Cortisol
Liver	↑ glucose output	↑↑↑ gluconeogenesis ↑ glycogenolysis ↑ ketogenesis	↑↑ gluconeogeneis ↑↑ ketogenesis ↑ glycogenolysis	↑ gluconeogenesis
Adipose tissue	↑ lipolysis ↓ glucose uptake	↑↑↑ lipolysis ↓ glucose uptake		↑ lipolysis
Muscle	↓ glucose uptake	↓ glucose uptake		↓ glucose uptake

- endocrine disease, e.g. Cushing's syndrome, acromegaly, Conn's syndrome, phaeochromocytoma;
- pancreatic tumours, e.g. glucagonoma, somatostatinoma; and
- genetic disorders, e.g. DIDMOD, MODY.

6.8 (a) T (b) F (c) F (d) T (e) F
Cholecalciferol is the natural form of vitamin D and the metabolism of this vitamin is as shown in Figure 6.2.

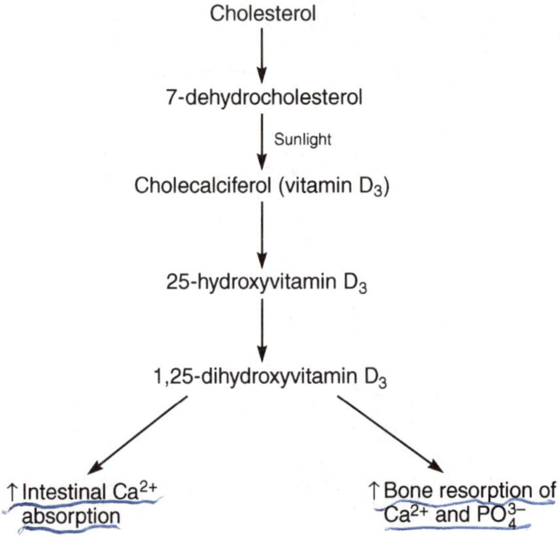

Figure 6.2 Metabolism of vitamin D.

The primary effect of 1,25-dihydroxyvitamin D is on the intestine. It also promotes the effect of parathyroid hormone on bone. Reduced plasma calcium concentration increases the formation of 1,25-dihydroxyvitamin D.

6.9 (a) T (b) F (c) F (d) T (e) T
Calcitonin is a polypeptide hormone secreted by parafollicular C-cells in the thyroid gland. An increase in plasma calcium concentration causes an increase in calcitonin secretion. Gastrointestinal hormones such as gastrin also stimulate secretion of calcitonin. The net effect of calcitonin is to reduce plasma calcium concentration by reduction of renal reabsorption of calcium and phosphate, and inhibition of resorption of bone.

6.10 (a) F (b) F (c) T (d) F (e) T

Phosphate metabolism is coupled with calcium metabolism though it is not quite as tightly controlled. Sixty to eighty per cent of ingested phosphate is absorbed from the intestine primarily by active transport processes. Some is also absorbed by passive diffusion. The major route by which phosphate is excreted is the kidney (15% of filtered phosphate). The principal site of phosphate reabsorption is the proximal tubule (70%). Parathyroid hormone exerts a major regulatory effect on phosphate excretion by inhibiting phosphate reabsorption in proximal tubules.

6.11 (a) T (b) F (c) F (d) F (e) F

To solve the problem of solubility and excessive urinary loss, thyroxine and steroid hormones rely on protein transporters. Specific carrier proteins include cortisol-binding globulin (cortisol and aldosterone), thyroxine-binding globulin (thyroxine [T4]), and sex-steroid binding globulin (testosterone and oestradiol).

These are specific and relatively high affinity carriers. Albumin is an important general carrier of steroid hormones and carries about 50% of circulating aldosterone and 10% of cortisol. Transthyretin carries thyroxine and some steroids and is a low affinity, non-specific carrier.

6.12 (a) T (b) F (c) F (d) T (e) F

Hormones can be characterized as belonging to one of three categories:

Amino acid derivatives:	adrenaline and noradrenaline from tyrosine melatonin from tryptophan thyroxine from tyrosine
Peptides or proteins:	**Peptides** thyrotrophin-releasing hormone parathyroid hormone growth hormone corticotrophic hormone (ACTH) follicle-stimulating hormone **Glycoproteins** follicle-stimulating hormone thyroid-stimulating hormone luteinizing hormone human chorionic gonadotrophin
Steroid hormones:	oestrogens, progesterone, testosterone, aldosterone.

6.13 (a) T (b) T (c) F (d) T (e) T

There are a number of mechanisms by which membrane receptors activate intercellular processes. Most receptors are glycoproteins with the sugar moieties on the extracellular surface. Protein hormones are hydrophilic and insoluble in the lipid layer of the plasma membrane. Membrane receptors rely on intracellular signalling mechanisms involving second messengers to produce their effects. Three second messenger systems have been identified:

1. adenylate cyclase/cyclic AMP system (eg. ACTH, glucagon, catecholamines);
2. phosphatidylinisotol and diacylglycerol systems; and
3. receptor-linked ion channels.

For some hormones such as insulin, receptors may be transmembrane proteins with a kinase region which phosphorylates intracellular proteins.

6.14 (a) F (b) F (c) T (d) F (e) T

Growth hormone is a 191-amino acid peptide hormone secreted by the anterior pituitary gland. Secretion is controlled by the hypothalamus (stimulated by growth hormone-releasing hormone and inhibited by somatostatin). Secretion is classically pulsatile in nature and peaks about 1 h after the onset of deep sleep. Rapid eye movement sleep returns secretion to normal levels. Growth hormone has a mixture of insulin-like and anti-insulin effects.

Muscle	**Liver**	**Adipose**
↑ amino acid uptake	↑ protein synthesis	↓ glucose uptake
↑ protein synthesis	↑ RNA synthesis	↑ lipolysis
↓ glucose uptake	↑ gluconeogenesis	
	↑ somatomedin production (insulin-like growth factors I and II)	

6.15 (a) F (b) T (c) T (d) F (e) F

The two primary regulators of aldosterone secretion are potassium ion concentration and angiotensin II (a peptide hormone). The kidneys play a key role in determining plasma levels of both of these factors and are also the major site of action. ACTH does not affect aldosterone secretion.

- Potassium ion increases of 5% increase aldosterone secretion.
- Renin is secreted in response to hypovolaemia. Renin, via effects on angiotensin I, ultimately leads to an increase in aldosterone secretion.

- Mineralocorticoids are secreted from the zona glomerulosa, glucocorticoids from the zona fasciculata and androgens from the zona reticularis.

6.16 (a) T (b) F (c) T (d) F (e) T

Glucocorticoids are transported mainly (80%) by corticosteroid-binding globulin, 15% by albumin and 5% is free. Steroid hormones are lipid-soluble and readily pass through the cell membrane and bind to receptors in the nucleus. Hormone receptor complexes then bind to specific sites on DNA, altering transcription of mRNA for specific proteins.

Effects of cortisol on metabolism

Liver
↑ gluconeogenesis
↑ glycogen synthesis

Skeletal muscle
↓ protein synthesis
↑ protein degradation
↓ glucose uptake

Adipose tissue
↓ glucose uptake
↑ lipid mobilization

6.17 (a) F (b) T (c) F (d) T (e) T

Blood lipids are transported by various lipoproteins. Chylomicrons transport mainly triglycerides derived from the diet. Triglycerides synthesized in the liver are transported mainly in VLDLs. Cholesterol derived from diet and liver synthesis is mainly carried in LDLs. High density lipoproteins carry cholesterol, derived from other tissues, to the liver. Cholesterol synthesis is controlled by HMGCoA reductase and this enzyme is inhibited by stains. Elevated concentrations of lipoproteins are found in some people with coronary heart disease. In people with heterozygous familial hypertriglyceridaemia, serum LDL cholesterol concentrations are elevated from birth, and, without treatment, over 50% of men die from coronary heart disease before the age of 60 years. Lipoprotein a is an independent risk factor for coronary heart disease and consists of the LDL particle linked to apo [a].

6.18 (a) T (b) T (c) T (d) F (e) F

In the first stage of glycolysis, glucose is phosphorylated to 1,6-fructose biphosphate. This consumes energy. Completion of glycolysis yields two molecules of pyruvic acid, a 3-carbon compound, releasing about 3% of the free energy ultimately obtained from glucose (two NADH and four ATP molecules).

The citric acid cycle contains a number of control points. When ATP is plentiful the cycle is slowed and when the supply of ATP is low it is accelerated. ATP is an allosteric inhibitor of citrate synthetase, reducing the formation of citrate. When ADP concentration rises (with lower ATP) isocitrate dehydrogenase is allosterically activated to increase production of α-ketoglutarate to speed up the cycle.

Oxidative phosphorylation by electron transfer via cytochromes generates 32 molecules of ATP. In total, glycolysis generates 36 ATP molecules, two from glycolysis, two from the citric acid cycle and 32 from oxidative phosphorylation in mitochondria.

High energy phosphate bonds in ATP have a free energy change (ΔG) for ATP → ADP + Pi of about –12 kcal/mol.

6.19 (a) T (b) F (c) F (d) F (e) T

During normal pregnancy the following hormones are secreted from the placenta:

- hCG maintains the corpus luteum and stimulates oestrogen and progesterone secretion; stimulates foetal gonad and adrenal synthesis of steroid hormones; and suppresses maternal lymphocytes.
- progesterone and oestrogen are essential for maintenance of endometrial growth and metabolism.
- human chorionic somatomammotrophin regulates maternal and foetal metabolism.

Maternal GnRH release is inhibited while prolactin, T3, T4 and aldosterone release is stimulated. Insulin secretion increases during the third trimester because of decreased maternal sensitivity to insulin.

In the second trimester the placenta takes up to 30% of maternal cardiac output.

6.20 (a) F (b) F (c) T (d) F (e) T

Vasopressin (ADH) is a nine-amino acid peptide secreted by the posterior pituitary gland. The primary effect is to increase water retention by the kidney, increasing blood and extracellular fluid volume. In addition to reducing urine volume it has a vasoconstrictor effect. The primary two stimuli to secretion are, first, an increase in blood or extracellular osmolality, and, second, a large decrease (>10%) in blood volume. Hypothalamic osmoreceptors are very sensitive to changes in osmolality and activate neuroendocrine cells of the supraoptic nucleus and trigger release of ADH. In addition to osmolality and blood volume, a number of other factors influence ADH secretion. Alcohol is a powerful inhibitor of ADH release. Nicotine, barbiturates and some anaesthetics stimulate ADH release. In neurogenic diabetes insipidus ADH levels are reduced but they are normal in nephrogenic diabetes insipidus.

6.21 (a) F (b) T (c) T (d) F (e) T
In 1994 a mouse obese (*Ob*) gene was sequenced and soon after a human homologue found. This gene codes for a protein called leptin and is expressed by adipocytes. Concentrations of leptin 'inform' the hypothalamus of the size of fat mass. Hypothalamic neuropeptide Y synthesis and release is inhibited by leptin, increasing food intake, insulin and corticosteroid levels in plasma. In animals and humans serum leptin concentrations are correlated with the size of fat mass but are not related to the development of non-insulin dependent diabetes mellitus.

6.22 (a) F (b) T (c) F (d) F (e) T

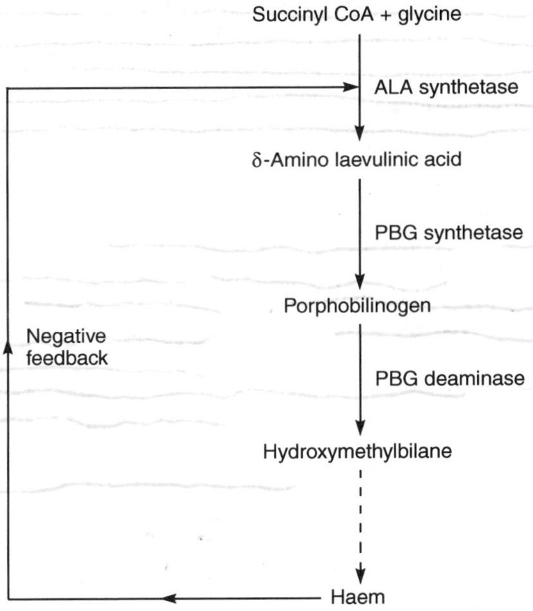

Figure 6.3 Enzyme pathway for haem production.

AIP is due to reduction in activity of PBG deaminase. Eleven mutations of the gene on the chromosome which produces PBG synthetase have been described. It is an autosomal dominant disorder and heterozygotes have 50% and homozygotes about 20% activity of PBG deaminase. It is more common in females and usually does not present until after puberty. The enzyme pathway for the production of haem is shown in Figure 6.3.

With reduced activity of PBG deaminase the normal inhibition of ALA synthetase by haem does not occur. Drugs which stimulate ALA synthetase drive the chain of reactions with accumulation of δ-ALA and PBG in the urine, and precipitation of an acute attack of AIP.

6.23 (a) T (b) T (c) T (d) T (e) F

The TSH-R is a prime autoantigen in Graves' disease and atrophic thyroiditis. These receptors are located on the basal surface of thyroid follicular cells. In Graves' disease autoantibodies stimulate the TSH-R, but have the opposite effect in autoimmune thyroiditis.

The TSH-R is a membrane receptor with transmembrane domains similar to the β_2 adrenergic receptor. Antibodies which bind to the TSH-R cross-react with heat shock protein 70 and to some gut micro-organisms.

Antibody levels tend to fall following treatment of Graves' disease and persistently high levels indicate that relapse is likely (60–100%). Carbimazole has its main anti-thyroid effect by reducing thyroid hormone synthesis by inhibition of iodinization and coupling. It also causes a reduction in TSH-R antibodies but does not affect the TSH receptor.

6.24 (a) T (b) F (c) F (d) F (e) T

T3 and T4 are synthesized from thyroglobulin (molecular weight 330 000) which is rich in tyrosine residues. Thyroid follicular cells iodinate tyrosine to produce mono- and di-iodothyronine. These are coupled to make T3 and T4. Both are insoluble and highly protein-bound, T3 (99.7%), T4 (99.9%). About 20% of T3 is made in the thyroid and the rest comes from peripheral conversion of T4 to T3. It is less tightly protein-bound and about four times more active. T3 and T4 enter cells largely by passive diffusion but some is also taken up by low and high affinity receptors. They both act by binding to nuclear receptors.

6.25 (a) T (b) F (c) T (d) F (e) F

The hypothalamus is crucial in neuroendocrine control. The posterior pituitary gland secretes vasopressin (ADH) and oxytocin. Both hormones are synthesized in the hypothalamus in the supraoptic and paraventricular nuclei, and are transported along axons to the posterior pituitary. Communication between the hypothalamus and the anterior pituitary is by the hypothalamic–pituitary portal system. Secretion of anterior pituitary hormones is under the control of several releasing/inhibiting hormones produced by the hypothalamus.

Hormone	**Action**
Corticotrophin RH (CRH)	ACTH secretion
Thyrotrophin RH (TRH)	TSH secretion
Gonadotrophin RH (GnRH)	LH and FSH secretion
Somatostatin	Inhibits GH secretion
Growth hormone RH (GRH)	Stimulates GH secretion
Prolactin releasing factor (PRF)	Stimulates prolactin secretion
Prolactin inhibitory factor (PIF) (dopamine)	Inhibits prolactin secretion

RH, releasing hormone.

FURTHER READING

Elder, G.H., Hift, R.J. and Meissner, P.N. (1997) The acute porphyrias, *Lancet*, **349**, 1613–17.

Greenspan, F.S. and Baxter, J.D. (1994) *Basic and Clinical Endocrinology*, Appleton and Lange, Connecticut.

Natrown, M. (1996) *Malins' Clinical Diabetes*. Chapman and Hall, London.

7 Respiratory medicine and cardiology

QUESTIONS

7.1 Alpha-1-protease inhibitor (α-1-antitrypsin):
(a) has a serum half-life of 4–5 days.
(b) is an important inhibitor of metalloproteases such as cathepsin G.
(c) deficiency causes clinical emphysema during the first decade of life.
(d) is very sensitive to oxidation by free radicals.
(e) therapy given intravenously is a routine treatment for deficient patients.

7.2 In pulmonary emphysema:
(a) there is a reduction in elastic recoil pressure.
(b) residual volume is decreased.
(c) diffusing capacity for carbon monoxide (D_LCO) is usually reduced.
(d) vital capacity is an accurate indicator of the extent of the disease.
(e) there is usually an improvement of 15% or more in FEV_1 following β_2-agonist treatment.

7.3 Nitric oxide (NO):
(a) is derived from L-arginine in airways epithelium.
(b) inhibits cholinergic bronchoconstriction *via* non-adrenergic, non-cholinergic (NANC) neural pathways.
(c) concentration is elevated in expired air in moderate to severe asthma.
(d) has a greater effect on airways smooth muscle compared to vascular smooth muscle.
(e) stimulates mucus secretion from submucosal glands.

7.4 The partial pressure of carbon dioxide (Pa_{CO_2}) in arterial blood:
(a) is measured indirectly from pH using the Astrup technique.
(b) can be assessed non-invasively by pulse oximetry.

(c) is usually elevated in a metabolic alkalosis.
(d) is often reduced in a metabolic acidosis.
(e) is elevated in lactic acidosis.

7.5 Diffusing capacity for carbon monoxide (D_LCO):
(a) is dependent on the volume of blood in the pulmonary capillaries.
(b) can be measured using open circuit spirometry.
(c) is increased in left to right shunts.
(d) is reduced in pulmonary emphysema.
(e) is a very specific test for the diagnosis of pulmonary fibrosis.

7.6 Risk factors in outbreaks of legionellosis include:
(a) water temperatures between 60 °C and 70 °C.
(b) generation of fine aerosols.
(c) high sugar content of water.
(d) the presence of limescale sludge.
(e) exposure of individuals with underlying lung disease.

7.7 Recognized factors in the pathogenesis of asthma include:
(a) cockroach allergy.
(b) rhinovirus infection in school age children.
(c) petrol fumes.
(d) activation of B cells.
(e) cat allergens.

7.8 The alveolar macrophage:
(a) has an important phagocytic role.
(b) is found in low numbers in bronchoalveolar lavage fluid.
(c) presents antigen to B lymphocytes.
(d) is a first line of cellular defence against mycobacteria.
(e) rarely releases chemotactic factors.

7.9 Ciliary function in the airways.
(a) may be impaired for up to 8 weeks by viral infection.
(b) is normal in Kartagener's syndrome.
(c) is dependent on myosin bridges between microtubules.
(d) is abnormal in patients with cystic fibrosis.
(e) is dependent on normal levels of secretory immunoglobulin A (IgA).

7.10 In the normal lung:
(a) there are four bronchopulmonary segments in the left lower lobe.
(b) the posterior segment of the right upper lobe is a frequent site of lung abscess.
(c) Clara cells secrete neuropeptides.
(d) ciliated epithelium secretes surfactant.
(e) bronchial walls have no submucosa.

7.11 The phrenic nerve:
(a) arises predominantly from the third cervical nerve.
(b) is a purely motor nerve.
(c) runs in front of the root of the lung.
(d) should be stimulated bilaterally with electrodes in quadriplegia with ventilatory failure.
(e) when paralysed unilaterally results in a 40% reduction in ventilation and perfusion of the lung on the affected side.

7.12 The following conditions commonly result in pulmonary function tests showing a reduced vital capacity and a normal transfer coefficient (KCO) for carbon monoxide:
(a) asbestosis.
(b) chronic asthma.
(c) extensive pleural disease.
(d) respiratory muscle weakness.
(e) fibrosing alveolitis.

7.13 The cystic fibrosis transmembrane conductance regulator (CFTR) protein:
(a) transports calcium ions.
(b) is present in skeletal muscle.
(c) has adenosine triphosphate (ATP) binding sites.
(d) is an intracellular molecule.
(e) conducts chloride ions in the presence of cyclic adenosine monophosphate (cAMP).

7.14 Amiodarone-induced pulmonary toxicity:
(a) only occurs at high doses of amiodarone.
(b) often presents with a cough as the only symptom.
(c) causes an obstructive defect on spirometry.
(d) causes giant cell formation in the airways mucosa.
(e) improves immediately amiodarone is discontinued.

7.15 During left ventricular systole:
(a) the left ventricle dilates before the aortic valve opens.
(b) the 'c' wave of jugular venous pressure is generated.
(c) the mitral valve ring descends.
(d) in aortic stenosis the phase of ejection is prolonged.
(e) in aortic regurgitation left ventricular output may be more than doubled.

7.16 In the coronary circulation:
(a) the right coronary artery usually supplies the atrioventricular node.
(b) the circumflex branch of the left coronary artery usually supplies the interventricular septum.
(c) blood from the left coronary artery is returned to the right ventricle mainly by anterior cardiac veins.
(d) blood in the coronary sinus is approximately 80% saturated with oxygen (Sa_{O_2}) in healthy individuals.
(e) blood flow occurs mainly during diastole.

7.17 Staphylococcal endocarditis:
(a) has a high mortality rate compared to other causes of endocarditis.
(b) is increasing in incidence.
(c) is a nosocomial infection in about 10% of cases.
(d) associated with *Staphylococcus lugdenensis* has a benign course.
(e) should be treated with parenteral antibiotics for 2 weeks.

7.18 Coronary artery tone is increased by:
(a) adenosine.
(b) thromboxane A_2.
(c) acetylcholine.
(d) α_2 receptor agonists.
(e) neuropeptide Y.

7.19 In the normal electrocardiogram:
(a) the normal QRS axis in the frontal plane is –60° to +30°.
(b) right axis deviation in the frontal plane is –30° to –90°.
(c) the normal QRS duration is 0.4 s.
(d) the QT interval is usually less than 0.12 s.
(e) the P wave is normally < 2 mm in height.

7.20 The following are recognized adverse effects of digoxin:
(a) atrioventricular junctional escape rhythms.
(b) mononeuritis multiplex.

(c) retrobulbar neuritis.
(d) hyperkalaemia.
(e) visual hallucinations.

7.21 Atrial natriuretic peptide (ANP):
(a) is secreted from the atria in response to stretching.
(b) decreases renal blood flow.
(c) decreases excretion of sodium.
(d) reduces secretion of aldosterone.
(e) levels are increased in congestive heart failure.

7.22 Endothelin 1:
(a) is generated by the action of endothelin-converting enzyme.
(b) causes smooth muscle contraction.
(c) functions primarily as a systemic hormone.
(d) levels in blood are reduced in chronic heart failure.
(e) generation is increased by hypoxia.

7.23 Adenosine:
(a) is a naturally occurring purine nucleoside.
(b) has a biological half-life of less than 1 min.
(c) stimulates specific myocardial receptors located in the atrioventricular node.
(d) is a recognized cause of bronchospasm.
(e) action is competitively inhibited by theophylline.

7.24 Familial (type IIa) hypercholesterolaemia:
(a) has an X-linked pattern of inheritance.
(b) is caused by a mutation of the gene for low density lipoprotein (LDL) receptors.
(c) usually results in coronary heart disease by the third decade of life.
(d) characteristically produces tendon xanthomata.
(e) is usually treated with 3-hydroxy,3-methylglutaryl co-enzyme A (HMGCoA) reductase inhibitors.

7.25 Neurohumoral changes in chronic cardiac failure include:
(a) increased arginine vasopressin (ADH).
(b) reduced endothelin.
(c) reduced atrial natriuretic peptide (ANP).
(d) elevated calcitonin gene-related peptide (cGRP).
(e) increased tumour necrosis factor alpha (TNFα).

ANSWERS

7.1 (a) T (b) F (c) F (d) T (e) F
α_1-antiprotease (α_1-PI) is a natural inhibitor of neutrophil elastase and other serine proteases. Inhibition is by irreversible binding. α_1-PI is in excess in serum and tissues. The body produces about 2 g/day and the serum half-life is 4–5 days. α_1-PI does not inhibit metalloproteases.

Deficiency of α_1-PI causes clinical emphysema during the third to fourth decade in smokers and later in non-smokers. It is associated with neonatal liver disease. α_1-PI is very sensitive to oxidative damage by free radicals. This is one of the mechanisms for lung disease in smokers. Studies are still on-going to determine whether intravenous replacement therapy is effective in deficient patients. Such therapy is not available in the UK but is in the USA and some European countries.

7.2 (a) T (b) F (c) T (d) F (e) F
Patients with pulmonary emphysema have reduced pulmonary compliance and elastic recoil pressure. Forced expiratory volume in one second (FEV_1) and vital capacity are usually reduced but the reduction in FEV_1 is greater. The lungs are overinflated with increased residual volume and total lung capacity. D_LCO and transfer coefficient (KCO) for carbon monoxide are usually reduced and give a broad indication of the extent of the disease. Vital capacity is not a good indicator of disease severity. It is uncommon to demonstrate significant reversibility to β_2 agonists in patients with emphysema.

7.3 (a) T (b) T (c) T (d) F (e) T
Nitric oxide (NO) is an important neurotransmitter and bronchodilator in the control of airways tone in healthy people. NO is a more 'powerful' vasodilator than bronchodilator. In inflammatory conditions such as asthma, increased NO production occurs because of inducible nitric oxide synthase (iNOs) from epithelial cells and macrophages. iNOs is induced by cytokines and oxidants and results in plasma leakage, mucus secretion and induction of T helper 2 (TH2) cells.

7.4 (a) F (b) F (c) F (d) T (e) F
The Pa_{CO_2} is measured using a direct recording electrode. The derivation of Pa_{CO_2} from pH (Astrup technique) is no longer in routine use. Pulse oximetry only measures oxygen saturation (Sa_{O_2}) and heart rate. Low Sa_{O_2} shifts the CO_2 content/Pa_{CO_2} dissociation curve to the left. The effects of acid–base disturbances on Pa_{CO_2} are as follows and depend on the equation:

$$CO_2 + H_2O \rightleftharpoons H_2CO_3 \rightleftharpoons HCO_3^- + H^+$$

In respiratory disorders, changes in the above equation are due to carbon dioxide while metabolic disorders change $[H^+]$ or $[HCO_3^-]$.

- Metabolic acidosis: $[H^+]$ increases, so the pH falls; $[HCO_3^-]$ falls, shifting the above equation to the left. The tendency for any rise in Pa_{CO_2} is more than offset by H^+ stimulation of the respiratory drive. Pa_{CO_2} is therefore reduced.
- Metabolic alkalosis: $[H^+]$ falls, so the pH rises; $[HCO_3^-]$ increases, shifting the above equation to the right. Increased Pa_{CO_2} tends to stimulate breathing and the pH has the opposite effect. The net effect is usually no change in Pa_{CO_2}.
- Respiratory acidosis: the increase in $[H^+]$ is secondary to increased Pa_{CO_2} and causes a shift to the right in the above equation. $[H^+]$ are buffered by proteins so the rise in $[HCO_3^-]$ may be more impressive than the $[H^+]$ rise.
- Respiratory alkalosis: $[H^+]$ falls because of overexcretion of CO_2, shifting the equation to the left.

7.5 (a) T (b) F (c) T (d) T (e) F

D_LCO is measured in a closed circuit with the patient inhaling gas with a low concentration of CO and helium. From this the 'transfer' of CO from the alveoli to the blood can be estimated. The D_LCO is dependent on the diffusing capacity of the membrane (D_m), the volume of blood in the pulmonary capillaries (V_c) and a constant representing gas uptake capacity per unit volume (θ) ($1/D_L = 1/D_m + 1/\theta V_c$).

D_LCO is elevated in polycythaemia, lung haemorrhage and left to right shunts (because of increased pulmonary blood volume).

D_LCO is reduced in, for example, emphysema, pulmonary fibrosis, extrapulmonary restriction, anaemia, pulmonary vascular disease, renal failure and cirrhosis. It is not a very specific test for any disease but is a sensitive test for abnormal pulmonary function.

7.6 (a) F (b) T (c) F (d) F (e) T

Legionellosis (Legionnaire's disease/Pontiac fever) is caused by *Legionella pneumophila* (14 serogroups). Infection is caused by respiratory aerosol usually spread from water in systems such as air conditioning. Risk factors in outbreaks include:

- Water temperature between 20 °C and 50 °C
- Growth nutrients (proteins and rust)
- Protected niches against biocides such as limescale
- Fine aerosolization of water

- Low water turnover
- Open to ingress of animals/dust/sunlight
- Susceptible individuals

7.7 (a) T (b) T (c) F (d) F (e) T

A large number of factors have been recognized in the pathogenesis of asthma (Figure 7.1). They play various roles in the causation of this condition. Cat and cockroach allergen are important inducers.

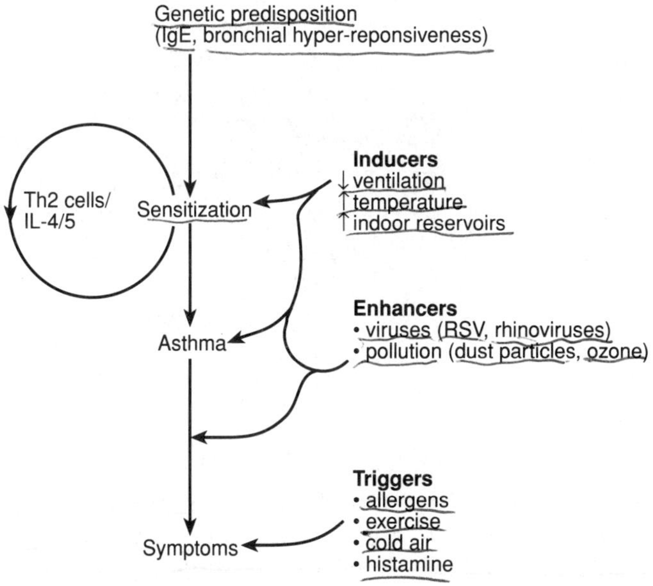

Figure 7.1 Pathogenesis of asthma.

7.8 (a) T (b) F (c) F (d) T (e) F

The alveolar macrophage is the most important and numerous phagocyte at the alveolar surface. It also has important effector cell functions modulating the activity of other inflammatory and immune responses. It has an important role as an antigen presentation cell (APC) to T lymphocytes and releases a large number of substances including cytokines, leukotrienes and complement factors. Macrophages are the predominant cell found in bronchoalveolar lavage fluid.

The important phagocytic role makes these cells the front line defence against respiratory pathogens such as tuberculosis.

7.9 (a) T (b) F (c) F (d) T (e) F

Ciliated epithelium is an important part of host defence mechanisms in healthy individuals and is found to the level of respiratory bronchioles. Cilia are similar to flagella found in bacteria and sperm tails. They usually beat at between 300 and 800 beats/min. The structure is as shown in Figure 7.2.

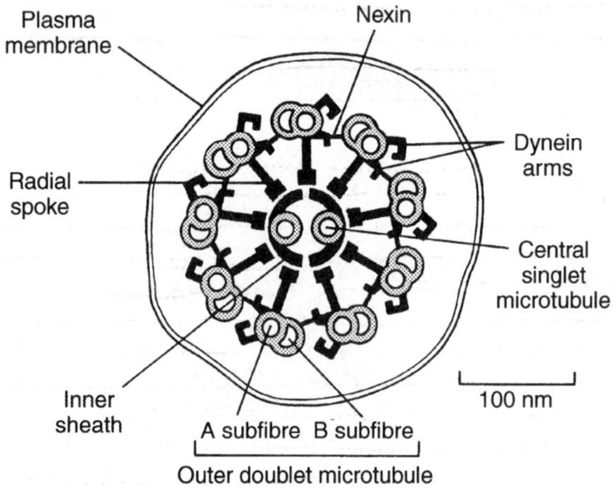

Figure 7.2 Structure of cilia.

Ciliary function may be impaired for up to 8 weeks by viral infections, such as influenza, which denude the epithelium. In cystic fibrosis exotoxins from bacterial infection impair ciliary clearance. A number of intrinsic ciliary disorders have been described. The absence of a dynein arm is a feature of Kartagener's syndrome. Ciliary function is independent of IgA secretion.

7.10 (a) T (b) T (c) F (d) F (e) F

Bronchopulmonary segments comprise the following:

- The upper lobe consists of three segments: apical, posterior and anterior (lingula superior and inferior on left).
- The middle lobe has two segments: medial and lateral (right only).
- The lower lobe can contain five segments: apical lower, anterior, lateral and posterior (plus medial on the right lung only).

The posterior segment of the right upper lobe is a frequent site for lung abscess formation (75%). Bronchi have a mucosa, submucosa and fibrocartilaginous layer. The mucosa is pseudostratified squamous epithelia set on an elastic lamina. Most of the mucosa is covered with ciliated epithelial cells. The following cells are found in the normal lung:

- Ciliated cells: there are 1500–2000/cm^2 and they are involved in mucociliary clearance.
- Goblet cells are found in larger airways, and secrete mucus.
- Clara cells secrete surfactant.
- Serous cells are secretory cells found in serous glands.
- Endocrine cells: amine precursor uptake and decarboxylation (APUD) cells, they are 5-hydroxytryptamine-positive.

7.11 (a) F (b) T (c) T (d) F (e) F

The phrenic nerve arises primarily from the fourth cervical root. The nerve runs through the mediastinum in front of the root of the lung. The right phrenic nerve is lateral to venous structures throughout its course. The left phrenic nerve runs lateral to the common carotid and left subclavian arteries, then lateral to the pericardium over the left ventricle. About two-thirds of phrenic nerve fibres are motor, the rest are sensory to the diaphragm, pleura and pericardium.

Paralysis of the phrenic nerve reduces the forced vital capacity and ventilation and perfusion by about 20% on that side.

In patients with quadriplegia stimulation of the phrenic nerve should be unilateral and on alternate sides every 6–8 h to stop fatigue of the diaphragm.

7.12 (a) F (b) T (c) T (d) T (e) F

Table 7.1 Pulmonary function tests in different conditions

	FEV_1	FVC	$D_{L}CO$	KCO
Asbestosis	↓	↓	↓	↓↓
Fibrosing alveolitis	↓	↓	↓	↓↓
Chronic asthma	↓↓	↓	↑ (sometimes)	↑ (sometimes)
Extensive pleural disease	↓	↓	↓	Normal or ↑
Respiratory muscle weakness	↓	↓↓	↓	Normal or ↑

In respiratory physiology, $D_{L}CO$ is the diffusing capacity for carbon monoxide and KCO is the transfer coefficient. FEV_1, forced expiratory volume in 1 s; FVC, forced vital capacity.

$D_{L}CO = KCO \times V_A$ (*V_A = alveolar volume*).

7.13 (a) F (b) F (c) T (d) F (e) T
CFTR protein is the product of the CFTR gene. Mutations of the gene (over 400 are described) if the individual is homozygous result in cystic fibrosis (i.e. the gene is recessive). CFTR is primarily a chloride ion channel but also partly controls sodium ion transport *via* effects on epithelial sodium channels (ENaC). The chloride ion channel is opened by cAMP. The protein is sited in the cell membrane with 12 transmembrane domains and intracellular nucleotide binding domain and an R domain with protein kinase A and C binding sites.

CFTR is expressed in epithelial cells, e.g. airways, skin, gut, vas deferens and biliary tract. It is not expressed in brain or muscle.

7.14 (a) F (b) F (c) T (d) F (e) F
Amiodarone is an effective anti-arrhythmic drug used in the management of atrial and ventricular dysrhythmias, particularly in patients with poor left ventricular function. It causes hepatic and thyroid dysfunction. Pulmonary toxicity occurs in less than 5% of patients and although it is more common in patients on doses over 400 mg/day can occur at lower doses. It often presents with non-specific symptoms of dyspnoea, cough, fever and weight loss. (Cough alone is a side effect of angiotensin-converting inhibitor therapy.) The chest radiograph usually demonstrates overinflation and a reticulonodular or 'ground glass' appearance, and pulmonary function tests usually show a predominantly obstructive pattern (though sometimes a mixed picture is seen). Lung damage is caused by toxic oxygen species and lung biopsies have increased lymphocytes, polymorphonuclear cells and 'foamy' macrophages. Toxicity is prolonged after discontinuation of the drug because of the long half-life of the drug. Oral corticosteroid treatment may be beneficial.

7.15 (a) F (b) F (c) T (d) T (e) T
During left ventricular systole the mitral valve closes and the pressure in the ventricle rises rapidly. The volume in the ventricle remains unchanged (isovolumetric contraction) until the aortic valve opens, followed by ejection of blood. This phase is prolonged in aortic stenosis. In aortic regurgitation the left ventricular output may be doubled.

During systole the mitral valve cusps move towards the left atrium, generating the 'c' wave following by the 'x' descent as the valve ring descends during aortic valve opening. The jugular venous pressure is generated by changes on the right side of the heart.

7.16 (a) T (b) F (c) F (d) F (e) T
The right coronary artery arises from the right coronary sinus of Valsalva and runs down the groove between the right atrium and ventricle. It usually supplies the sinus node, atrioventricular node and bundle, the right ventricle and posterior part of the left ventricle. The left coronary artery arises from the left coronary sinus of Valsalva and divides into the anterior descending (LAD) and circumflex branch. The LAD supplies the interventricular septum and the anterior wall of the left ventricle. The circumflex supplies the lateral and posterior aspects of the left ventricle. Blood flow in the coronary circulation mainly occurs during diastole.

The coronary sinus drains blood from the left ventricle and the anterior cardiac veins drain the right anterior right ventricular wall. Oxygen extraction by cardiac muscle is high so coronary sinus blood has an Sa_{O_2} of < 40%.

7.17 (a) T (b) T (c) T (d) F (e) T
Staphylococcal endocarditis is a serious condition associated with high morbidity and mortality rates. The incidence of staphylococcal endocarditis is increasing and accounts for about 50% of cases of bacterial endocarditis. Between 10 and 20% of cases are associated with organisms acquired in hospital, often because of infection of intravenous catheters. *S. lugdenensis* is a recently described coagulase-negative organism causing endocarditis and is associated with rapid destructive disease. Emergency valve replacement may be required. Treatment for staphylococcal endocarditis should be for at least 2 weeks using an anti-staphylococcal penicillin and an aminoglycoside combination.

7.18 (a) F (b) T (c) F (d) T (e) T
Coronary artery smooth muscle contains α, β_1, dopamine and parasympathetic receptors. A large number of vasoactive substances can change coronary artery tone:

Vasoconstrictors	**Vasodilators**
α_2 receptor agonists	Ischaemic myocardium, e.g. adenosine, lactate, H^+ and bradykinin
Dopamine (>15μg/kg/min)	β-receptor agonists ($\beta_1 > \beta_2$)
Cold pressor test	dopamine < 5μg/kg/min
Ergot alkaloids	Parasympathetic receptors
Thromboxane A_2	Acetylcholine
Prostaglandin F	Ca^{++} antagonists
Neuropeptide Y	Prostaglandin E
	cGRP, vasoactive intestinal polypeptide (VIP) and substance P

7.19 (a) F (b) F (c) F (d) F (e) T
The normal QRS axis in the frontal plane is –30° to +90°. The axis of electrical deflections can be determined on the hexaxial reference system, as shown in Figure 7.3.

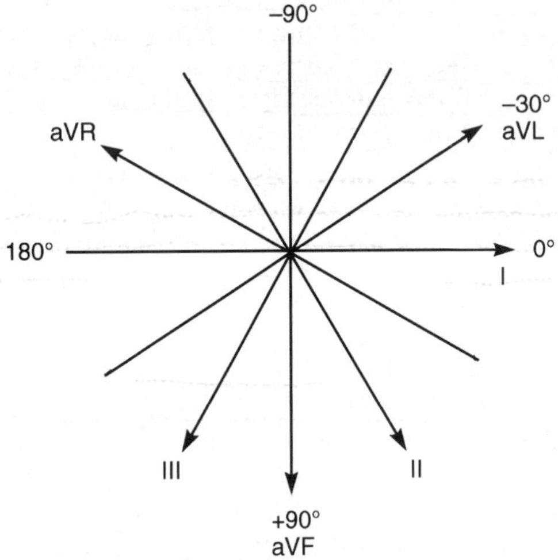

Figure 7.3 Hexaxial reference system.

Left axis deviation is –30° to –90°. Right axis deviation is +90° to 180°. Deflections of –90° to 180° indicate extreme right or left axis deviation. Normal intervals follow:

- PR 0.2 s
- QRS 0.1 s
- Q < 0.04 s wide (and < 25% of QRS complex)
- QT interval must be corrected for heart rate
- QTc = QT = 0.38 s.

7.20 (a) T (b) F (c) T (d) T (e) T
The incidence of digoxin toxicity is 10–20% and predominantly affects the heart, central nervous system (CNS), eye and gut.

Cardiac:	Almost any dysrhythmia, most commonly ventricular extra beats, bigeminy, atrioventricular rhythms, heart block, VT and atrial fibrillation.

CNS:	Headache, fatigue, confusion and visual hallucinations.
Visual:	Blurred vision, halos, xanthopsia (yellow vision) and retrobulbar neuritis
Gastrointestinal tract	Nausea, vomiting and anorexia.
Others:	Hyperkalaemia, particularly in overdose because of inhibition of Na+/K^+ pumps. [K^+] > 5.5 mmol/l is an indication for anti-digoxin anti-body fragments.

7.21 (a) T (b) F (c) F (d) T (e) T

ANP is a polypeptide hormone released following atrial distension, leading to a diuresis and natriuresis. Renal blood flow is increased and by interaction with the renin angiotensin system aldosterone production is reduced. The homeostatic function of ANP is to control circulatory blood volume by opposing sodium and water retention. In congestive heart failure, ANP levels are elevated but are insufficient to overcome the hormonal and circulatory forces leading to fluid retention.

7.22 (a) T (b) T (c) F (d) F (e) T

Endothelin 1 is a vasoconstrictor and pressor peptide generated by endothelial cells, and has an important role in the maintenance of basal vascular tone and arterial blood pressure. It is released as 'big' endothelin 1 and the active form is generated by endothelin-converting enzyme. Endothelin acts on type A receptors on smooth muscle cells. Vasoconstriction is modulated by type B receptors which cause vasodilatation by the actions of nitric oxide and prostacyclin. Although endothelin 1 is present in the plasma and may generally influence vascular tone its primary action is paracrine on smooth muscle cells. Endothelin 1 is increased by a wide range of vasoactive and inflammatory mediators, physical circulatory factors and hypoxia. Endothelin 1 is elevated in chronic heart failure and is a good predictor of survival. Endothelin receptor antagonists may have a role in the treatment of cardiac failure.

7.23 (a) T (b) T (c) F (d) T (e) T

Adenosine is a nucleoside formed in the body by serial dephosphorylation of adenosine triphosphate (ATP). The biological half-life is very short, of the order of 1.5 to 10 s. Adenosine receptors are present in myocardial cells (A1), endothelium and vascular smooth cells (A2). A rapid injection causes a fall in blood pressure by 10–15 mmHg followed by a transient increase. There is also a biphasic effect on heart rate.

When given intravenously, adenosine does not cause bronchoconstriction but does so when given by nebulizer. Theophylline and caffeine are competitive antagonists of adenosine.

7.24 (a) F (b) T (c) T (d) T (e) T

Familial hypercholesterolaemia is an autosomal dominant disorder involving a mutation of the gene for LDL receptors. The heterozygous form affects about 1 in 500 Caucasian people. Tendon xanthomas, corneal arcus and xanthelasma are common and males usually develop coronary artery disease in their fourth or fifth decades. Total cholesterol and LDL cholesterol levels are usually double the acceptable levels. Treatment almost always should include an HMGCoA reductase inhibitor.

7.25 (a) T (b) F (c) F (d) F (e) T

The net effect of circulating neurohumoral changes in chronic cardiac failure is to increase systemic vascular resistance. The following neurohumoral systems are activated, causing vasoconstriction:

- Sympathetic nervous systems (adrenaline and noradrenaline)
- Increased endothelin
- Renin/angiotensin axis
- Aldosterone
- Neuropeptide Y
- Vasoconstrictor prostaglandins.

Parasympathetic activity and endothelial-dependent vasodilatation are reduced, as are circulating concentrations of cGRP. TNFα concentrations are elevated.

A number of compensatory vasodilators are elevated, such as dopamine, ANP and vasodilator prostaglandins.

FURTHER READING

Berne, R.M. and Levey, M.N. (1992) *Cardiovascular Physiology*, Mosby – Year Book.

Gibson, G.J. (1992) *Clinical Tests of Respiratory Function*, Raven Press, New York.

Lundberg, J.O.N., Lundberg, J.M., Alving, K. and Wentzberg, E. (1997) Nitric oxide and inflammation. *Nat Med*, **3**, 30–1.

Penningtown, J.E. (1994) *Respiratory Infections*, Raven Press, New York.

Platts-Mills, T.A.E. and Carter, M. (1997) Asthma and indoor pollution. *N Eng J Med* **336**, 1382–3.

Priebe, H.J. and Skarvan, K. (1995) *Cardiovascular Physiology*, BMJ Publishing, Plymouth.

Wilkins, M.R. *et al.* (1997) The natruiretic peptide family, *Lancet*, **349** 1307–10.

8 Renal, liver and gastrointestinal medicine

QUESTIONS

8.1 Loop diuretics (e.g. frusemide):
(a) principally act on the thick, ascending limb of the lop of Henlé.
(b) inhibit basolateral sodium/potassium ATPases.
(c) can cause allergy in patients sensitive to sulphonamides.
(d) cause greater hypokalaemia than thiazide diuretics.
(e) promote calcium loss.

8.2 In the renal circulation:
(a) normally 40–50% of the cardiac output is taken.
(b) arteriolar tone is adjusted to maintain flow when blood pressure falls.
(c) vascular tone is maintained by circulating catecholamines.
(d) vascular tone is the highest in the glomerular capillary.
(e) vasoconstriction of the efferent arteriole results in a fall in glomerular filtration rate (GFR).

8.3 The proximal renal tubule:
(a) is the site where the majority of filtered sodium is reabsorbed.
(b) reabsorbs some sodium ions co-transported with organic solutes.
(c) is a site of action of carbonic anhydrase inhibitors.
(d) epithelial membrane has a low permeability for water.
(e) epithelial cells have an important sodium/potassium ATPase (Na^+/K^+ ATPase) on their lumenal membranes.

8.4 Renin:
(a) is a low molecular weight polypeptide hormone.
(b) is produced by renal cortex cells.
(c) converts angiotensin I to angiotensin II.
(d) secretion is reduced by reduced solute concentrations (Na^+ or Cl^-) to the distal convoluted tubule.
(e) secretion is increased by atrial natriuretic peptide (ANP).

8.5 When renal function is normal:

(a) the tubular maximum reabsorptive capacity for phosphate ($TmPO_4$) is often exceeded under normal physiological conditions when dietary phosphate is increased.

(b) the $TmPO_4$ is increased by parathyroid hormone.

(c) aldosterone stimulates potassium secretion by cortical collecting ducts.

(d) systemic alkalosis leads to potassium retention by the kidney.

(e) carbenoxolone administration causes increased potassium excretion in the urine.

8.6 The following diuretics and their primary sites of renal action are linked correctly:

(a) mannitol: thin, descending loop of Henlé.

(b) frusemide: thick, ascending limb of loop of Henlé.

(c) metolazone: early, distal tubule.

(d) bendrofluazide: proximal tubule.

(e) spironolactone: collecting duct.

8.7 In glomerulonephritis:

(a) antibodies to glomerular basement membrane (GBM) occur in about 25% of cases.

(b) T cell activation is associated with aggressive disease.

(c) associated with anti-neutrophil cytoplasmic antibodies (ANCA) there is invariably linear immunoglobulin G (IgG) deposition.

(d) associated with acute hepatitis B infection immune complexes of HBs, HBe and HBc antigens are found in the GBM.

(e) associated with Henoch–Schölein purpura (HSP), there is usually immunoglobulin A (IgA) deposition in the mesangium.

8.8 Sodium reabsorption from tubular fluid in the nephron is:

(a) linked with glucose reabsorption in the distal tubule.

(b) accompanied by water reabsorption in the loop of Henlé.

(c) reduced by amiloride.

(d) increased in the distal tubule in the nephrotic syndrome.

(e) an important determinant of the osmolality of medullary interstitial fluid.

8.9 Renal actions of prostaglandins include:

(a) inhibition of renin release.

(b) inhibition of adenylate cyclase in tubular and ductal cells.

(c) stimulation of anti-diuretic hormone (ADH)-mediated fluid retention.

(d) vasodilatation when noradrenaline levels are elevated.
(e) increased potassium excretion.

8.10 Inability to lower the urine pH below 5.2 is a characteristic feature of:
(a) cranial diabetes insipidus.
(b) chronic lithium therapy.
(c) cystinosis.
(d) respiratory failure.
(e) chronic pyelonephritis.

8.11 The following statements regarding liver drug metabolism are correct:
(a) lipid-soluble drugs usually have a higher first metabolism than water-soluble drugs.
(b) P450 enzymes are situated on smooth endoplasmic reticulum.
(c) hepatocellular carcinoma is associated with long-term use of C17-substituted testosterone.
(d) paracetamol toxicity occurs when liver glutathione stores are depleted.
(e) omeprazole is an inducer of P450 enzymes.

8.12 Bilirubin:
(a) when unconjugated, is water-soluble.
(b) is all derived from haemoglobin.
(c) uridine diphosphate (UDP) glucuronyl transferase is elevated in Gilbert syndrome.
(d) diglucuronide passively diffuses into biliary cannaliculae.
(e) in Crigler–Najjar syndrome is unconjugated.

8.13 The following statements about ethanol metabolism are true:
(a) ethanol is oxidized by alcohol dehydrogenase in hepatocytes.
(b) acetaldehyde levels in blood are elevated in chronic alcoholism.
(c) paracetamol and alcohol compete for the same P450 enzyme.
(d) ethanol is used to synthesize free fatty acids in the liver.
(e) ethanol induces gamma-glutamyl transpeptidase (γGTP).

8.14 Kupffer cells:
(a) are derived from hepatocytes.
(b) remove denatured proteins from the circulation.
(c) have specific receptors for the Fc portion of immunoglobulin.
(d) form a continuous wall of the sinusoid.
(e) when activated, secrete tumour necrosis factor-α.

8.15 The following statements regarding pancreatic digestive enzymes are correct:

(a) they are most active at pH 7.4.
(b) they are released in response to cholecystokinin.
(c) they include a deoxyribonuclease.
(d) lipase is important in the conversion of triacylglycerols to monoglycerides and free fatty acids.
(e) trypsinogen is converted to trypsin by secretin.

8.16 Bile salts are:

(a) essential for cholesterol excretion in bile.
(b) reabsorbed from the terminal ileum.
(c) present in plasma in highest concentration shortly before a meal.
(d) synthesized from cholesterol.
(e) often present in plasma in increased amounts in patients with cirrhosis.

8.17 Gastric parietal cells:

(a) secrete a solution of hydrochloric acid (HCl) of pH 3.
(b) are stimulated by gastrin to secrete gastric acid.
(c) are the most abundant cells found in gastric epithelium.
(d) secrete intrinsic factor.
(e) contain carbonic anhydrase for the production of HCl.

8.18 Gastric H^+/K^+ ATPase (proton pump):

(a) is located in tubulovesicles in parietal cells.
(b) consists of alpha and beta sub-units.
(c) binds omeprazole covalently to its alpha sub-unit.
(d) is found in other tissues.
(e) is an autoantigen in pernicious anaemia.

8.19 *Campylobacter jejuni*:

(a) is a Gram-positive organism.
(b) is the most common organism isolated in enteric infections.
(c) infection is rarely associated with systemic symptoms.
(d) infections are frequently associated with poultry ingestion.
(e) infections can be treated with fluoroquinolone antibiotics.

8.20 The following statements regarding the digestion and absorption of oligosaccharides are true:

(a) fructose is absorbed by passive diffusion.
(b) digestion requires the presence of normal small intestinal villi.
(c) glucose absorption is coupled with sodium.

(d) glucose absorption requires the expenditure of metabolic energy.
(e) the major disaccharide produced from amylase digestion of starch is maltose.

8.21 Triacylglycerols (TAGs):
(a) are hydrophilic.
(b) are emulsified in the small intestine by bile salts.
(c) are a major component of micelles.
(d) account for about 90% of dietary fat intake.
(e) are a major constituent of chylomicrons.

8.22 *Helicobacter pylori*:
(a) infects approximately 20% of individuals over 50 years.
(b) causes gastro-oesophageal reflux disease (GORD).
(c) produces urease.
(d) is associated with low plasma gastrin levels.
(e) causes a strong humoral immune response in man.

8.23 The following statements regarding gastrointestinal hormones are correct:
(a) motilin increases gastric motor activity.
(b) somatostatin decreases gastric secretion.
(c) pancreatic polypeptide stimulates pancreatic bicarbonate secretion.
(d) enteroglucagon decreases the small bowel transit rate.
(e) secretin maintains mucosal growth.

8.24 Histological features in the colon which favour a diagnosis of Crohn's disease rather than ulcerative colitis include:
(a) the formation of pseudopolyps.
(b) involvement of rectal mucosa.
(c) crypt abscess formation.
(d) eosinophilia of the submucosa.
(e) Langerhan's giant cells.

8.25 Obesity:
(a) is defined as a body mass index (BMI) of over 25 kg/m^2.
(b) affects about 10% of the population.
(c) can be due to Laurence–Moon–Biedl syndrome.
(d) results in an increased mortality rate from digestive diseases compared to that in lean individuals.
(e) is associated with an increased incidence of cardiovascular disease.

ANSWERS

8.1 (a) T (b) F (c) T (d) F (e) T

Loop diuretics act on the ascending loop of Henlé by interfering with the apical co-transporter which mediates the entry of sodium from the lumenal fluid into this segment (1K^+, 1Na^+, 2Cl^-). This leads to loss of these ions and water. Frusemide and bumetanide contain –SO_2NH_2 sulphonamide groups in common with thiazides and carbonic anhydrase inhibitors and can cause sulphonamide allergy. Diuretics acting on the distal tubule are non-sulphonamides (e.g. amiloride, spironolactone). Loop diuretics cause less potassium loss compared to thiazides, probably because of their shorter duration of action. Loop diuretics cause loss of calcium while thiazides increase calcium reabsorption.

8.2 (a) F (b) T (c) F (d) F (e) F

At rest the renal circulation accounts for 20–25% of cardiac output. Changes in systemic blood pressure result in rapid and at times dramatic changes in arteriolar pressure in order to maintain a normal GFR. Resistance vessels, the afferent and efferent arterioles, control this process. Vasoconstriction of these vessels causes the following effects: a fall in GFR and renal blood flow (RBF) in the afferent arteriole, and a rise in GFR and fall in RBF in the efferent arteriole.

Tone is controlled *via* the juxtamedullary apparatus and not systemic vasoconstrictor hormones. Glomerular capillary pressure is about 45 mmHg.

8.3 (a) T (b) T (c) T (d) F (e) F

The proximal renal tubule is the site of 65–80% of sodium reabsorption, together with corresponding anions and water. The epithelium of the proximal tubule is very permeable to water. A number of mechanisms control reabsorption of sodium.

- Basolateral (not lumenal) Na^+/K^+ ATPases.
- Co-transport with organic solutes accounts for a small amount of Na^+ transport.
- Bicarbonate transport via a carbonic anyhydrase Na^+/H^+ exchanger accounts for about 20% of sodium transport.
- Electrochemical and physical fluxes (solvent drag) also account for some Na^+ transport.

8.4 (a) F (b) F (c) F (d) F (e) F

Renin is manufactured in juxtaglomerular cells as pro-renin which is a large molecular weight peptide and is converted intracellularly to its active form of renin which is a serine protease of molecular weight 40 000. It is important in the renin–angiotensin cascade as illustrated in Figure 8.1.

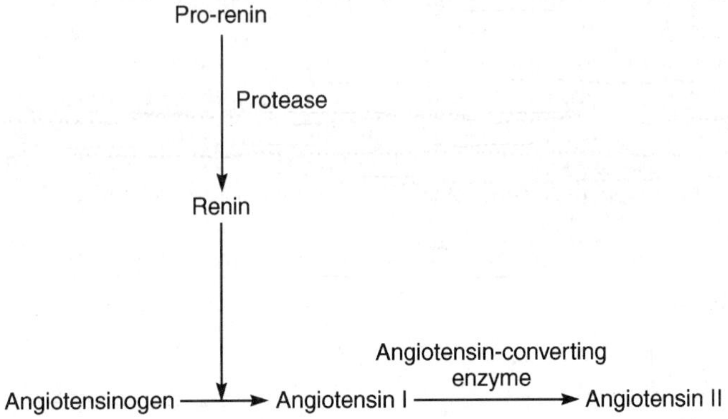

Figure 8.1 Renin–angiotensin cascade.

Renin release is increased by:

- reduced renal arteriolar pressure
- reduced delivery of solute to the distal convoluted tubule
- increased sympathetic nervous system activity
- high $[K^+]$ in the plasma.

Renin secretion is inhibited by:

- angiotensin II
- ANP
- vasopressin.

8.5 (a) T (b) T (c) T (d) F (e) T

The tubular transport maximum (Tm) for substances is an expression of the limited reabsorptive capacity of the tubules. If the Tm is exceeded, loss of the substance in the urine occurs. When renal function is normal the $TmPO_4$ is close to the filtered phosphate load and phosphate is usually excreted when dietary intake increases. Parathyroid hormone inhibits phosphate reabsorption by increasing the $TmPO_4$

Acidosis in the body is initially buffered by bicarbonate. Hydrogen ions are then excreted in the urine combined with urinary buffers such as inorganic phosphate and ammonia.

When renal function is normal and plasma levels of potassium are normal or elevated, potassium is secreted by cortical collecting ducts.

The following cause urinary potassium wasting: alkalosis, hyperaldosteronism (e.g. Conn's syndrome, carbenoxolone ingestion), Cushing's syndrome and hypomagnesaemia.

8.6 (a) F (b) T (c) T (d) F (e) T

Mannitol is an osmotic which interferes with sodium absorption in proximal and distal tubules by entraining water in the tubule. The site of action of other diuretics is shown in Table 8.1.

Table 8.1 Site of action of diuretics

Site of action	Drug	Mechanism
Proximal tubule	Carbonic anhydrase inhibitors	Blocks H^+ for apical Na^+/H^+ exchanger
Thick ascending limb of loop of Henlé	'Loop' diuretics	Blocks $Na^+/K^+/2Cl^-$ co-transporter
Early distal tubule	Thiazides	Blocks Na^+/Cl^- co-transporter
Late distal tubule/ cortical collecting duct	Sodium channel blockers (amiloride/triamterene)	Blocks apical Na^+ channel
	Aldosterone antagonists	Blocks aldosterone receptor

8.7 (a) F (b) T (c) F (d) T (e) T

Glomerulonephritis (GN) may be initiated by the following immune stimuli: autoimmunity to glomerular antigens (e.g. anti-GBM disease); endogenous extra-renal antigens (e.g. autoimmune disease and tumour antigens) and exogenous antigens (e.g. microbial products, drugs and foreign serum).

Anti-GBM disease is uncommon, causing < 5% of cases of GN. Cell injury in GN is caused by deposited antibody, complement components, cytokines, eicosonoids and coagulation factors. In addition, cell-mediated responses are important and activated T cells are associated with aggressive disease. Linear IgG deposition is associated with anti-GBM disease, granular IgG with immune complex disease and sparse glomerular immune reactants with ANCA-associated vasculitis. Acute hepatitis B infection can cause acute GN (usually in children) and is associated with hepatitis B antigen–antibody complex deposition. HSP is associated with IgA deposits in the mesangium.

8.8 (a) F (b) F (c) F (d) T (e) T

Sodium concentration in intracellular fluid is kept within narrow limits. It is freely filtered by the glomerulus and 99% is reabsorbed by the tubular system.

Around 70–80% of sodium resorption occurs in the proximal tubule. The active transport mechanism is driven by basolateral Na^+/K^+ ATPase. The proximal pathways on the luminal surface include: co-transport with glucose, sodium/hydrogen exchanger, chloride flux causes an electrochemical gradient for sodium and solvent drag.

The loop of Henlé is where 25% of sodium resorption occurs, but it is impermeable to water. Transport relies on a $Na^+/K^+/Cl^-$ lumenal transporter and a basal Na^+/K^+ ATPase.

About 5–8% of sodium resorption takes place in the distal tubule. Sodium chloride is reabsorbed by an electroneutral co-transporter. The basolateral membrane has a Na^+/K^+ ATPase.

8.9 (a) F (b) T (c) T (d) T (e) F

The kidney synthesizes prostaglandins from the prostanoid group (PGE_2, $PGF_{2\alpha}$, $PGPI_2$ and thromboxane). Arachidonic acid is also released from lipid membranes. PGE_2 is the predominant renal prostaglandin. Renal actions of prostaglandins are outlined below:

- actions on blood flow, opposing angiotensin and adrenergic vasoconstriction
- renal sodium excretion
- tubular adenylate cyclase inhibition opposing ADH effects
- stimulation of renin release.

Prostaglandins have no effect on potassium excretion. Cyclooxygenase inhibitors (e.g. non-steroidal anti-inflammatory drugs) cause a fall in renal blood flow and glomerular filtration rate, and salt and water retention because of their effects on prostaglandin metabolism.

8.10 (a) F (b) T (c) T (d) F (e) T

The inability to acidify urine is a feature of renal tubular acidosis (RTA). RTA is defined as systemic metabolic acidosis because of a specific tubular abnormality, often out of proportion to the degree of renal impairment. There is usually hyperchloraemia and urine pH is greater than 5.7. RTA associated with bicarbonate wasting is usually proximal RTA. Causes of distal RTA are genetic/idiopathic, autoimmune disorders (e.g. systemic lupus erythematosus, chronic active hepatitis and Sjögren's syndrome), nephrocalcinosis (e.g. primary hyperparathyroidism or medullary sponge kidney), tubulointerstitial disease (e.g. chronic pyelonephritis and renal transplants) and drugs (e.g. analgesics, lithium, amphotericin B).

Proximal RTA (bicarbonate wasting) is caused by Fanconi syndrome, cystinosis, Wilson's disease, tubulointerstitial diseases, drugs and amyloidosis.

There is a third group of RTA associated with hyperkalaemia and hypoammonuria.

8.11 (a) T (b) T (c) T (d) T (e) T

Liver clearance of drugs depends on the efficiency of metabolizing enzymes, first pass effect, liver blood flow and extent of protein binding.

Drugs which are avidly taken up by the liver have a high first pass metabolism and are usually lipid-soluble compounds. P450 enzymes (haemoproteins) are mostly associated with smooth endoplasmic reticulum and include over 50 enzymes. Those involved in drug metabolism are in groups I–III. Examples of inducers are omeprazole (P450Ia1), ethanol (IIE1) and rifampicin (IIIA).

Paracetamol is metabolized to its toxic metabolite which is inactivated by glutathione. Hepatic necrosis occurs when glutathione is depleted.

8.12 (a) F (b) F (c) F (d) F (e) T

Bilirubin is the end product of haem, myoglobin and cytochrome enzyme metabolism. About 80% of bilirubin is derived from haem. Unconjugated bilirubin is insoluble and is tightly bound to albumin. A small amount is dialysable and this amount increases when bilirubin is displaced by drugs such as sulphonamides. The liver extracts bilirubin–albumin complexes by specific carrier proteins. Albumin is recycled and the bilirubin conjugated by bilirubin UDP glucuronyl transferase to a monoglucuronide and diglucuronide. Reduced concentrations of this enzyme cause the hyperbilirubinaemia associated with Gilbert syndrome and neonatal jaundice. Bilirubin diglucuronide is actively excreted into the bile cannaliculi against the concentration gradient. Crigler–Najjar syndrome is a familial non-haemolytic hyperbilirubinaemia associated with very high levels of unconjugated bilirubin. It can be autosomal recessive or dominant and is because of absent, or greatly reduced function of, glucuronyl transferase.

8.13 (a) T (b) T (c) T (d) F (e) T

Alcohol cannot be stored in the body so all of it is oxidized. This mostly takes place in the cytosol but some is also metabolized in mitochondria by P450 enzymes (microsomal ethanol oxidizing system).

The P450 IIE1 has a high affinity for ethanol and drugs such as paracetamol. The metabolism of alcohol is shown in Figure 8.2.

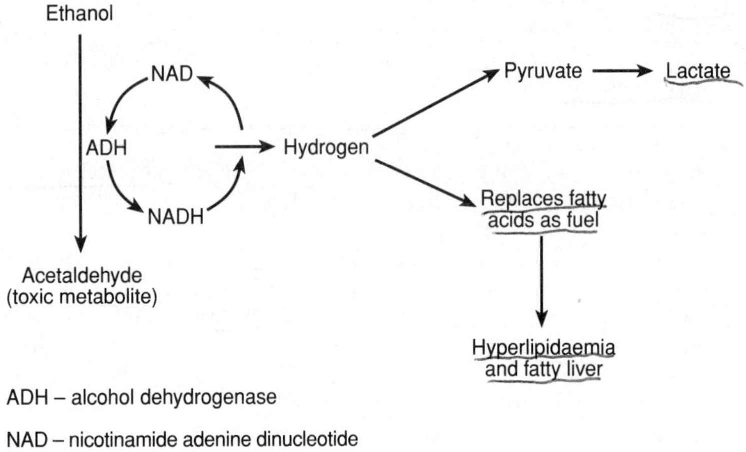

Figure 8.2 Metabolism of alcohol.

Acetaldehyde is a toxic metabolite and may injure hepatocytes by peroxidation, superoxide formation and stimulation of collagen synthesis. Levels of this metabolite may be elevated in chronic alcoholism. Ethanol induces γGTP, giving rise to elevated blood levels.

8.14 (a) F (b) T (c) T (d) F (e) T

Kupffer cells are derived from monocytes and function as phagocytes in the liver. They endocytose micro-organisms, tumour cells and proteins. They have specific receptors for the Fc portion of immunoglobulin and the C3b component of complement. They are important antigen-presenting cells. When activated they secrete cytokines such as tumour necrosis factor alpha, and interleukins and prostaglandins. Endothelial cells line the lumen of the sinusoid.

8.15 (a) T (b) T (c) T (d) T (e) F

Pancreatic secretion is made up of bicarbonate which is actively secreted by intercalated ductal cells. This is dependent upon carbonic anhydrase. Enzymes are secreted by acinar cells. Cholecystokinin released from the duodenal mucosa (when fat or protein comes into contact with it) stimulates secretion of pancreatic enzymes and

Table 8.2 Function of digestive enzymes

Enzyme		Action/products
Proteolytic		
Trypsinogen →	Trypsin ↓	Proteins to peptides
Chymotrypsinogen	→ chymotrypsin	
Procarboxypeptidase	→ carboxypeptidase	Cleaves carboxyl group amino acids
Carbohydrate		
Amylase		Polysaccharides to oligosaccharides
Lipolytic		
Lipase		Triacylglycerides to monoglycerides and free fatty acids
Phospholipase		Lecithin to fatty acid and lysolecithin
Cholesterol esterase		Cholesterol esters to free fatty acids and cholesterol
Nucleolytic		
Ribonuclease		Nucleic acids to mononucleotides
Deoxyribonuclease		

secretin stimulates bicarbonate secretion. The function of digestive enzymes is outlined in Table 8.2.

8.16 (a) T (b) T (c) F (d) T (e) F
Bile salts are synthesized from cholesterol by hepatocytes and are actively transported into bile cannaliculi. Liver bile is 97% water, and around 1% each of bile pigments and salts. Gallbladder bile has less water (15%). Food entering the small intestine causes release of cholecystokinin which stimulates contraction of the gallbladder and relaxation of the sphincter of Oddi. Bile salts play an important role in rendering monoglycerides and free fatty acids water-soluble with the formation of micelles. Bile salts traverse the small intestine and are actively reabsorbed in the terminal ileum. They are then removed from the blood by hepatocytes and recycled (enterohepatic circulation). Bile salts are at their highest concentration in portal blood during a meal and are in low concentration between meals when they are stored in the gallbladder. Patients with chronic liver disease have a deficiency of bile salts because of impaired synthesis.

8.17 (a) F (b) T (c) F (d) T (e) T
Gastric parietal cells secrete HCl with a hydrogen ion concentration $[H^+]$ of 150 mmol/l (pH 0.9). This is 3×10^6 the $[H^+]$ of blood and

requires ATP to move H^+ and Cl^- against the concentration gradient. Carbonic anhydrase is important in the production of H^+ from water and carbon dioxide. Parietal cells release HCl by neuronal stimulation *via* acetylcholine (cephalic phase) and hormonal stimulation by gastrin (gastric phase). Both of these mechanisms are probably locally mediated by histamine. Gastric parietal cells secrete intrinsic factor. Chief cells which secrete pepsinogen are the most abundant cells in gastric epithelium.

8.18 (a) T (b) T (c) T (d) T (e) F
The H^+/K^+ ATPase is a member of the family of phosphorylating ion transport ATPases. It consists of an α and β sub-unit. The pumps are made in the smooth endoplasmic reticulum and transported *via* tubovesicles to the cannaliculi of the parietal cell where they insert into the cell membrane and become functional.

Omeprazole covalently binds with cysteines found in the α sub-unit of the pump.

There are various proton pumps present in mammalian cells such as the multimeric mitochondrial and vacuolar pumps.

8.19 (a) F (b) T (c) F (d) T (e) T
C. jejuni and other campylobacters are the most common organisms isolated in enteric infections. Campylobacters are small Gram-negative rods. They have a single polar flagellum. Infection is usually associated with direct contact with animals, including pets. Poultry is particularly implicated but other meat products can be contaminated. Campylobacter infection usually presents with systemic symptoms of malaise, fever, abdominal pain and diarrhoea. In severe cases a fulminant colitis has been described. Treatment is indicated in severe cases and fluoroquinolone may be useful in reducing faecal excretion and duration of symptoms.

8.20 (a) T (b) T (c) T (d) T (e) T
Starch is the major carbohydrate in the human diet and is digested by amylase to maltose, a disaccharide containing two glucose molecules. Other fragments containing between five and nine glucose molecules (oligosaccharides) are also produced. Oligosaccharides are hydrolysed to monosaccharides by disaccharidases (e.g. maltase, lactase and sucrase) at the microvilli brush border.

Fructose is absorbed by facultative diffusion, while glucose and galactose are actively transported into the portal circulation by a carrier-mediated process located in the brush border. This is coupled with sodium co-transport.

8.21 (a) F (b) T (c) F (d) T (e) T

TAGs account for about 90% of dietary lipid intake. They are very hydrophobic. Pancreatic lipase and bile salts are required for absorption. When TAGs enter the small intestine they are in the form of large droplets. These are emulsified by bile salts and this increases the number of molecule of TAGs available to lipase for digestion to monoglycerides and free fatty acids. These products of digestion with bile salts form micelles. These small aggregates contain about 20 molecules and are important as a reservoir to allow absorption of individual fat molecules into epithelial cells. Cholesterol and fat-soluble vitamins undergo a similar process of absorption. Following absorption, monoglycerides and free fatty acids are reconstituted to form TAGs in epithelial cell smooth endoplasmic reticulum. A phospholipid layer is added to each droplet of TAG aggregates to form a chylomicron, which enters the lacteal of the villus.

8.22 (a) F (b) F (c) T (d) F (e) T

Helicobacter pylori is a spiral micro-aerophilic, flagellated Gram-negative organism. It produces urea to maintain a relatively alkaline microenvironment in the stomach mucosa. Approximately 50–60% of individuals over the age of 50 years are infected. Infection causes mucosal inflammation and depletion of somatostatin stored in D cells of antral mucosa. This removes the normal inhibitory control over release of gastrin from G cells. The ensuing hypergastrinaemia stimulates parietal cells to hypersecrete hydrochloric acid and damage duodenal mucosa.

H. pylori infection plays a crucial role in the development of duodenal ulcers and has a lesser but important role in gastric ulceration. It is less clear whether it causes non-ulcer dyspepsia. There is no evidence of a role in gastro-oesophageal reflux disease.

The diagnosis of *H. pylori* may be made from serology as it induces a brisk humoral immune response. Urea breath tests and antral mucosal biopsy can also be used for diagnosis.

8.23 (a) T (b) F (c) F (d) F (e) F

Motilin, 22-amino acid residue peptide, is secreted by duodenal mucosa and is responsible for stimulating gastric and duodenal activity.

Gastrin stimulates gastric motility and secretion.

Somatostatin increases gastric activity but inhibits histamine release in response to gastrin and so reduces gastric secretion.

Secretin is the most powerful hormonal stimulus to pancreatic bicarbonate secretion.

Cholecystokinin also stimulates pancreatic secretion and synergizes with secretin. Pancreatic polypeptide inhibits bicarbonate secretion.

Neurotensin, peptide YY and enteroglucagon are neurohormonal markers for the small bowel and have potential roles in inhibiting gastric acid secretion, but their physiological significance is unclear.

8.24 (a) F (b) F (c) F (d) T (e) T

Crohn's disease most commonly involves the terminal ileum and right side of the colon. In contrast, ulcerative colitis almost always involves the rectum. The macroscopic appearance of Crohn's disease includes strictures, 'skip' lesions and cobblestone appearance.

Pseudopolyps are a feature of ulcerative colitis. The microscopic features in the two disorders are as follows:

Ulcerative colitis	**Crohn's disease**
Mucosal/submucosal inflammation	Transmural inflammation
No granulomas	Granulomas present (Langerhan's giant cells, eosinophilia)
Crypt abscesses common, loss of goblet cells	Crypt abscesses infrequent, normal goblet cell numbers
Pseudopolyp formation	Arteritis, pseudopyloric gland metaplasia

8.25 (a) F (b) T (c) T (d) T (e) T

Obesity is defined as a BMI of greater than 30 kg/m^2 in males or 28 kg/m^2 in females. In the latest census this means that about 8% of males and 12% of females in the UK have a BMI of greater than 30.

Obesity is only rarely associated with a clear genetic defect, e.g.

- Laurence–Moon–Biedl syndrome is an autosomal recessive disorder (obesity, mental handicap and retinitis pigmentosa).
- Prader–Willi syndrome (diabetes mellitus, hyptonica and mental handicap).
- Hypothalamic disease and some endocrine disorders (e.g. myxoedema and Cushing's disease) are associated with obesity.

Obesity is associated with a higher mortality rate from cardiovascular disease, diabetes mellitus and digestive disorders (colorectal, biliary and stomach cancers).

FURTHER READING

Bouchier, A.D., Allan, R.N., Hodgson, H.J.F. and Keighley, M.R.B. (1993) *Gastroenterology, Clinical Science and Practice*, WB Saunders, London.

Godwin, C.S. (1997) *Helicobacter pylori* infection, *Lancet*, **349** 265–9.
Sherlock, S. and Dooley, J. (1993) *Diseases of the Liver and Biliary System*, Blackwell Scientific Publications, London.
Whitworth, J.A. and Lawrence, J.R. (1994) *Text Book of Renal Disease*, Churchill Livingstone, Edinburgh.

9 Neuroanatomy and neurophysiology

QUESTIONS

9.1 The following statements are true:

(a) complete division of the optic tract results in unilateral blindness.
(b) a lesion of the optic chiasm may cause a homonymous hemianopia.
(c) a pituitary adenoma may cause a bitemporal upper quadrantanopia.
(d) retrobulbar neuritis is a recognized cause of bitemporal hemianopia.
(e) thrombosis of the anterior cerebral artery may result in a homonymous hemianopia.

9.2 The oculomotor (III) nerve:

(a) has no sensory component.
(b) passes through the cavernous sinus.
(c) innervates the superior oblique muscle.
(d) is responsible for elevation of the upper eyelid.
(e) may be compressed by an anterior communicating artery aneurysm.

9.3 A lesion affecting the facial nerve within the facial canal may cause:

(a) loss of taste over the anterior two-thirds of the tongue.
(b) hyperacusis.
(c) loss of cutaneous sensation over the cheek.
(d) ptosis.
(e) inability to blink on the affected side.

9.4 The left recurrent laryngeal nerve:

(a) is a branch of the vagus nerve.
(b) has motor and sensory components.
(c) innervates the cricothyroid muscle.
(d) innervates the upper one-third of the oesophagus.
(e) if sectioned, results in paralysis of both abductors and adductors of the left vocal cord.

9.5 Section of the posterior interosseous nerve will result in:
(a) paralysis of brachioradialis.
(b) paralysis of abductor pollicis brevis.
(c) paralysis of extensor pollicis longus.
(d) paralysis of extensor indicis.
(e) loss of cutaneous sensation over most of the dorsal aspect of the hand.

9.6 The consequences of a lesion affecting the median nerve at the elbow include:
(a) loss of pronation of the forearm.
(b) inability to flex the interphalangeal joints of the index and middle fingers.
(c) wasting of the hypothenar eminence.
(d) inability to oppose the thumb and forefinger.
(e) loss of sensation over the medial aspect of the palm.

9.7 The following statements are true:
(a) adductor pollicis is innervated by the ulnar nerve.
(b) the dorsal interossei are innervated by the radial nerve.
(c) all muscles of the hypothenar eminence are innervated by the ulnar nerve.
(d) the lumbricals are all innervated by the median nerve.
(e) opponens pollicis is innervated by the median nerve.

9.8 Clinical findings comparable with an injury of the common peroneal nerve include:
(a) paralysis of gastrocnemius.
(b) paralysis of dorsiflexion and eversion of the ankle.
(c) paralysis of toe extension.
(d) loss of sensation over the sole of the foot.
(e) an absent plantar response.

9.9 The following reflexes and their segmental levels are correctly paired:
(a) triceps – T1.
(b) knee jerk – L4.
(c) cremasteric – L2.
(d) plantar – S1.
(e) supinator – C6.

9.10 The following structures are involved in the light reflex:
(a) lateral geniculate body.
(b) Edinger–Westphal nucleus.
(c) abducent (VI) nerve.
(d) ciliary ganglion.
(e) nucleus ambiguus.

9.11 Regarding the adult spinal cord:
(a) the spinal cord has 30 pairs of spinal nerves.
(b) the C8 nerve root exits from the neural foramen below the eighth cervical vertebra.
(c) the cord terminates at the level of the first lumbar intervertebral disc.
(d) the great anterior medullary artery (of Adamkewicz) is the major blood supply to the upper third of the cord.
(e) a lesion of an anterior nerve root will result in sensory loss to the area it supplies.

9.12 The following modalities of sensation are conveyed in the dorsal columns of the spinal cord:
(a) proprioception.
(b) light touch.
(c) pain.
(d) vibration.
(e) temperature.

9.13 A lesion in:
(a) both frontal lobes is associated with a sucking reflex.
(b) both temporal lobes may be associated with cortical blindness.
(c) the angular gyrus of the dominant parietal lobe is associated with inability to read (alexia).
(d) the optic tract in the occipital lobe will abolish the pupillary light reflex on that side.
(e) Broca's area is associated with receptive aphasia.

9.14 The posterior inferior cerebellar artery:
(a) is a branch of the vertebral artery.
(b) supplies the medulla oblongata.
(c) supplies the vestibular nucleus.
(d) if occluded, may be associated with ipsilateral Horner's syndrome.
(e) if occluded, typically results in ipsilateral facial weakness.

9.15 Cerebrospinal fluid (CSF):
(a) opening pressure at lumbar puncture is normally 7–18 mmHg.
(b) normally contains up to 10 neutrophils per mm^3.
(c) immunoglobulin A (IgA) levels are higher than those in plasma.
(d) has a lower pH than plasma.
(e) is produced at a rate of approximately 500 ml/day.

9.16 Regarding neurons:
(a) dendrites conduct impulses towards the cell body.
(b) Golgi type I neurons have long axons.
(c) neurotransmitters are synthesized in the cell body and transported along the axon to the nerve terminal.
(d) most neurons do not contain mitochondria.
(e) the Nissl substance synthesizes neurotransmitters.

9.17 The following statements are correct:
(a) the resting membrane potential of a neuron is approximately +70 mV.
(b) during depolarization of an axon there is a rapid flux of potassium ions into the cell.
(c) influx and efflux of ions during the action potential is an active process.
(d) the refractory period is dependent on the length of the neuron.
(e) inhibitory stimuli cause influx of chloride ions.

9.18 Regarding excitation and conduction in neurons:
(a) the action potential is always an 'all-or-nothing' response.
(b) a decrease in the extracellular calcium concentration decreases the excitability of neurons.
(c) conduction velocity increases along the axon.
(d) conduction velocity increases with fibre diameter.
(e) conduction velocity is greater in myelinated than in unmyelinated neurons.

9.19 The following are recognized neurotransmitters in the central nervous system:
(a) muscarine.
(b) 5-hydroxytryptophan.
(c) L-dopa.
(d) glutamate.
(e) gamma-aminobutyric acid.

9.20 The following statements are correct:
(a) the synthesis of acetylcholine (ACh) is catalysed by acetylcholinesterase.
(b) noradrenaline is formed by the hydroxylation of dopamine.
(c) the principal mode of inactivation of ACh is by reuptake into the presynaptic terminal.
(d) serotonin is a derivative of tyrosine.
(e) monoamine oxidase is located in the synaptic cleft.

9.21 Regarding acetylcholine receptors:
(a) receptors at all autonomic ganglia are muscarinic.
(b) receptors at the skeletal neuromuscular junction are nicotinic.
(c) nicotinic receptors can be selectively blocked by atropine.
(d) M_2 muscarinic receptors mediate a negative chronotropic effect.
(e) pilocarpine is a muscarinic agonist.

9.22 Regarding neurons in the central nervous system:
(a) most fibres are myelinated.
(b) dorsal root C fibres convey sensations of pain and temperature.
(c) gamma motor neurons only innervate muscle spindles.
(d) postganglionic sympathetic fibres are unmyelinated.
(e) type Ia fibres to the muscle spindle have annulospiral endings.

9.23 In a spinal reflex arc:
(a) cell bodies of afferent neurons are located in the dorsal root ganglia.
(b) type Ib fibres convey afferent impulses from the Golgi tendon organ.
(c) type Ia fibres convey afferent impulses from the muscle spindle.
(d) flexor and extensor reflexes of the same limb cannot be made to contract simultaneously.
(e) evoking a flexor reflex in one limb will cause extension of the opposite limb.

9.24 Regarding the autonomic nervous system:
(a) sympathetic preganglionic neurons leave the spinal cord with the dorsal roots of spinal nerves T1–L3.
(b) most postganglionic neurons are unmyelinated.
(c) all preganglionic neurons are cholinergic.
(d) the hypoglossal nerve carries preganglionic parasympathetic fibres to the sublingual gland.
(e) sympathetic postganglionic neurons innervating sweat glands are classified as noradrenergic.

9.25 Regarding the electroencephalogram (EEG):
(a) alpha rhythm is abolished when the eyes are open.
(b) slow waves are always abnormal in an alert adult.
(c) a 3-Hz spike wave pattern is characteristic of subacute sclerosing panencephalitis.
(d) Creutzfeldt–Jakob (CJD) disease and the new variant (nvCJD) have an identical EEG pattern.
(e) absent EEG activity is required in order to diagnose brain death in the UK.

ANSWERS

9.1 (a) F (b) T (c) T (d) F (e) F

The optic chiasma is located above the pituitary fossa and is formed by the fibres from the nasal halves of each retina decussating to the opposite optic tract. Temporal fibres pass through the chiasm without decussating. Upper fibres of the radiation convey information from the lower part of the visual field and pass through the parietal lobe; the lower fibres convey information from the upper visual field, and pass through the temporal lobe.

A complete lesion of one optic tract causes a homonymous hemianopia. Damage to the temporal fibres of the optic radiation results in a homonymous upper quadrantanopia. Injury to the fibres in the parietal lobe results in a homonymous lower quadrantanopia.

Bitemporal hemianopia is most commonly caused by a suprasellar pituitary adenoma compressing the optic chiasm. Pressure on the lower fibres of the chiasm by an expanding pituitary tumour may cause a bitemporal upper quadrantanopia. Less frequently, pituitary tumours may exert pressure asymmetrically on the optic chiasm to cause a homonymous hemianopia. The posterior cerebral artery supplies most of the optic radiation and its occlusion may result in a homonymous hemianopia. Retrobulbar neuritis presents with painful, rapid loss of vision over 2–3 days. Lesions of the optic nerve cause unilateral blindness.

9.2 (a) T (b) F (c) F (d) T (e) F

The oculomotor nerve is entirely motor. It has two nuclei in the midbrain: the main motor nucleus which lies at the level of the superior colliculus, and the accessory parasympathetic nucleus (Edinger–Westphal nucleus). The nerve emerges from the anterior aspect of the midbrain and travels forward between the posterior cerebral artery and the superior cerebellar artery, passes through the lateral wall of the cavernous sinus (along with the trochlear (IV), maxillary and ophthalmic nerves), and enters the orbit through the superior orbital fissure. The oculomotor nerve supplies the levator palpebrae superioris and all external ocular muscles except the lateral rectus (VI) and superior oblique (IV). Preganglionic parasympathetic fibres synapse in the ciliary ganglion and pass *via* the short ciliary nerves to the constrictor pupillae and ciliary muscles, causing pupillary constriction and accommodation of the eye. A single central nucleus controls levator palpebrae superioris bilaterally, such that a complete lesion of the oculomotor nucleus results in bilateral ptosis. The oculomotor nerve may be compressed by aneurysms of the posterior communicating or posterior cerebral arteries, resulting in painful, total third nerve palsy with a dilated unreactive pupil. The abducent (VI) nerve passes through the cavernous sinus.

9.3 (a) T (b) T (c) F (d) F (e) T

The facial nerve enters the internal auditory meatus with the vestibulocochlear nerve and passes through the facial canal. As it descends in the facial canal it gives rise to the nerve to stapedius and the chorda tympani nerve (containing taste fibres from the anterior two-thirds of the tongue) before emerging from the stylomastoid foramen. The facial nerve divides into its five terminal branches within the substance of the parotid gland and supplies all of the muscles of facial expression. The facial nerve also carries parasympathetic secretomotor fibres to the lacrimal, submandibular and sublingual salivary glands. Complete interruption of the facial nerve at the stylomastoid foramen paralyses all muscles of facial expression. Painful sensitivity to loud sounds (hyperacusis) results if the nerve is damaged proximal to the origin of the nerve to stapedius. Division of the cervical sympathetic chain paralyses the smooth muscle of the levator palpebrae superioris, causing ptosis.

9.4 (a) T (b) T (c) F (d) F (e) T

The recurrent laryngeal nerves are branches of the vagus nerves: the right recurrent laryngeal nerve loops below the subclavian artery and ascends behind the carotid sheath between the oesophagus and trachea; the left loops below the ligamentum arteriosum between the aortic arch and pulmonary trunk, and passes behind the aorta to ascend between the oesophagus and trachea. Each nerve is closely associated with the inferior thyroid artery on each side, making it vulnerable to damage during thyroid surgery. Each nerve enters the larynx behind the cricothyroid joint and supplies all the intrinsic muscles of the larynx, except the cricothyroid muscles (innervated by the external laryngeal nerve, a branch of the superior laryngeal nerve), and also innervates the mucous membranes of the pharynx and larynx below the level of the cords. Complete section of one of the recurrent laryngeal nerves results in paralysis of the vocal cord in the midposition between abduction and adduction. The oesophagus is innervated by the vagus nerve.

9.5 (a) F (b) F (c) T (d) T (e) F

The radial nerve (C5–8) supplies the muscles of the extensor compartment of the arm and forearm, with a variable cutaneous supply. The radial nerve divides into its two terminal branches at the level of the lateral epicondyle of the humerus, into the superficial and deep radial nerves. The deep branch passes through the substance of the supinator muscle and emerges as the posterior interosseous nerve. This descends between the superficial and deep extensor muscles with the posterior interosseous artery and terminates on the back of the carpus. The posterior interosseous nerves supplies the extensor digitorum, extensor indicis, extensor digiti minimi, extensor carpi ulnaris, extensor pollicis longus and brevis, and abductor pollicis longus.

Brachioradialis is supplied by the radial nerve; abductor pollicis brevis is supplied by the median nerve. Section of the superficial branch of the radial nerve may only result in sensory loss over a small area over the dorsum of the hand, in the web between the thumb and index finger.

9.6 (a) T (b) T (c) F (d) T (e) F

The median nerve (C5–8, T1) in the forearm supplies the pronator muscles and the long flexor muscles of the wrist and fingers. A lesion at the elbow results in the arm being held in the supine position; wrist flexion is weak, and there is a degree of adduction because of unopposed action of the flexor carpi ulnaris and the medial half of flexor digitorum profundus (both innervated by the ulnar nerve). The index and middle fingers are incapable of flexion at the interphalangeal joints, though weak flexion of the metacarpophalangeal joints of these fingers is possible by the interossei. In attempting to make a fist, the index and middle fingers remain straight while the ring and little fingers flex (but are weakened by the loss of the lateral half of flexor digitorum superficialis). Paralysis of flexor pollicis longus results in inability to flex the distal phalanx of the thumb, which becomes laterally rotated and adducted. The muscles of the thenar eminence are paralysed and the eminence becomes flattened.

The median nerve supplies cutaneous sensation to the lateral half of the palm, the palmar aspect of the lateral three and a half fingers, and to the distal parts of the dorsal surfaces of these digits. The muscles of the hypothenar eminence are innervated by the ulnar nerve.

9.7 (a) T (b) F (c) T (d) F (e) T

The small muscles in the hand supplied by the median nerve are: the lateral two *L*umbricals, *O*pponens pollicis, *A*bductor pollicis brevis and *F*lexor pollicis brevis (LOAF).

The remaining small muscles (adductor pollicis, palmaris brevis, medial two lumbricals, all palmar and dorsal interossei, and the muscles of the hypothenar eminence) are innervated by the ulnar nerve (C7, 8, T1). The small muscles of the hand are innervated by the C8/T1 roots of the median and ulnar nerves.

9.8 (a) F (b) T (c) T (d) F (e) F

The common peroneal nerve (L4,5, S1,2), the smaller, lateral branch of the sciatic trunk, innervates the anterior and lateral compartments of the leg. After supplying the lateral head of biceps femoris in the popliteal fossa, it enters the calf by passing behind the head of the fibula and divides into the superficial and deep peroneal nerves. The superficial peroneal nerve supplies the peroneus longus and brevis muscles, terminating distally as cutaneous branches to the dorsum of the foot. The deep peroneal nerve supplies extensors digitorum longus and brevis, peroneus tertius, extensor hallucis longus and tibialis anterior. Injury to the common peroneal nerve results in paralysis of dorsiflexion and eversion (foot drop) and toe extension.

The tibial nerve (L4,5, S1–3), the larger division of the sciatic trunk, supplies popliteus, soleus, gastrocnemius, tibialis posterior, flexor digitorum longus and flexor hallucis longus. Its terminal branches supply the small muscles of the sole of the foot, and cutaneous sensation to the sole of the foot. Damage to the tibial nerve results in inability to plantar-flex or invert the foot, inability to flex the toes, inability to stand on the ball of the foot, and loss of sensation over the sole.

The sciatic nerve is composed of the common peroneal and tibial nerves. Section of the sciatic nerve results in loss of all movement below the knee, and loss of the ankle jerk.

9.9 (a) F (b) T (c) T (d) T (e) T

Tendon reflexes		**Superficial reflexes**	
Biceps	C5/6	Plantar	L5, S1
Supinator	C5/6	Abdominal	T7–12
Triceps	C7/8	Cremasteric	L1/2
Finger flexors	C8	Bulbocavernosus	S3/4
Quadriceps	L3/4	Anal	S3/4
Gastrocnemius	S1/2	Scapular	C5–T1

Primitive reflexes	
Glabellar	Corticopontine
Snout	Corticopontine
Sucking	Frontal
Palmomental	Frontal
Grasp	Frontal
Jaw	Pons

Myotomes	
C5	Deltoid
C6	Biceps
C7	Triceps
C8	Finger flexors
L3	Quadriceps
L5	Extensor hallucis longus
S1	Plantar flexors

9.10 (a) F (b) T (c) F (d) T (e) F

When a light is shone in one eye, afferent impulses pass through the optic nerve, optic chiasm and optic tract. Before reaching the lateral geniculate body, a small number of fibres leave the tract and pass to the pretectal nucleus, which sends fibres to synapse in the Edinger–Westphal nuclei on the ipsilateral and contralateral sides. Impulses then travel via parasympathetic fibres in the oculomotor nerve to the ciliary ganglion in the orbit. Postganglionic parasympathetic fibres then pass to the constrictor pupillae *via* the short ciliary nerves, causing pupillary constriction (direct light reflex). Since the pretectal nucleus sends fibres to both Edinger–Westphal nuclei, the contralateral pupil also constricts (consensual light reflex). The nucleus ambiguus, situated in the medulla, is the common motor nucleus of the glossopharyngeal (IX), vagus (X) and accessory (XI) nerves.

9.11 (a) F (b) T (c) T (d) F (e) F

The spinal cord has 31 pairs of spinal nerves, arising from anterior (motor) and posterior (sensory) nerve roots: eight cervical, 12 thoracic, five lumbar, five sacral and one coccygeal. Cervical roots (except C8) exit from neural foramina above their respective vertebral bodies. The C8 root emerges between C8 and T1. Thoracic and lumbar roots exit below each vertebral body. The spinal cord receives its blood supply from anterior and posterior spinal arteries (branches of the vertebral arteries), and from segmental spinal arteries (anterior and posterior radicular arteries). The great anterior medullary artery of Adamkewicz arises unilaterally from the aorta, usually entering the spinal cord from the left; it may be the principal blood supply to the lower two-thirds of the cord. The cord terminates at the level of the first lumbar intervertebral space (i.e. between L1 and L2) in adults, and at the level of L3 in children.

9.12 (a) T (b) F (c) F (d) T (e) F

Sense	**Central pathway**
Pain	Lateral spinothalamic
Temperature	Lateral spinothalamic
Light touch and pressure	Anterior spinothalamic
Discriminatory touch	Dorsal columns
Vibration	Dorsal columns
Joint position	Dorsal columns

Pain and temperature impulses travel to the spinal cord in fast conducting delta A fibres, and slow conducting C fibres which synapse with cells of the substantia gelatinosa before crossing over and ascending in the lateral spinothalamic tract. The sensations of light touch and pressure ascend in the anterior spinothalamic tract. The sensations of discriminatory touch, vibratory sense and joint position sense are carried in long ascending neurons in the posterior columns (fasciculus cuneatus and fasciculus gracilis) which ascend ipsilaterally to synapse with second order neurons in the nuclei gracilis and cuneatus in the medulla oblongata. The fasciculus gracilis contains fibres from the sacral, lumbar and lower six thoracic spinal nerves; the fasciculus cuneatus contains fibres from the upper six thoracic and all the cervical spinal nerves.

9.13 (a) T (b) T (c) T (d) F (e) F

Lesions of the motor and premotor areas of the **frontal lobes** result in contralateral spastic paralysis and contralateral grasp and palmomental reflexes. Bilateral lesions may be associated with a sucking reflex. Lesions of the prefrontal cortex are associated with abnormal social behaviour and altered personality. Lesions of Broca's motor speech area, in the inferior frontal gyrus, are associated with expressive aphasia.

Hearing is represented bilaterally in the superior surface of the **temporal lobe** (Heschl's gyri). Lesions of the optic tract (from the inferior retina) result in a contralateral homonymous upper quadrantanopia. Bilateral lesions of this pathway cause cortical blindness; pupillary reflexes are unaffected. Lesions of Wernicke's speech area in the superior convolution of the dominant lobe results in receptive aphasia. Lesions of the amygdaloid nucleus and hippocampus may result in loss of retentive memory; bilateral lesions may lead to excessive aggression.

The postcentral convolution of the **parietal lobe** serves somatic sensation for the opposite side of the body. Painful, tactile and thermal stimuli often return after injury to this area, but sensory discrimination (two point discrimination, stereognosis and localization of sensory stimuli) may remain impaired. The deep white matter contains fibres of the optic tract (from the upper retina), and lesions may result in a contralateral homonymous lower quadrantanopia. Lesions of the angular gyrus of the dominant hemisphere cause inability to read (alexia). The parietal lobe is important in the perception of one's position in space, the relationship of parts of the body to one another, and to other objects.

The **occipital lobe** contains the visual cortex: lesions of the optic tract cause a homonymous hemianopia. Visual illusions and hallucinations may also occur. Bilateral lesions result in cortical blindness. Injury to the area of visual cortex directly above the calcarine sulcus will cause a contralateral homonymous lower quadrantanopia; lesions in the area below the sulcus cause a homonymous upper quadrantanopia. Lesions in the dominant hemisphere may result in visual agnosias.

9.14 (a) T (b) T (c) T (d) T (e) F

The posterior inferior cerebellar artery is the largest branch of the vertebral artery. The proximal segment supplies the lateral medulla and the spinal tract and nucleus of the trigeminal nerve, the spinothalamic tract and nucleus ambiguus. Its distal branches supply the inferior aspect of the cerebellum and vermis. It also supplies the choroid plexus of the fourth ventricle. The lateral medullary syndrome may result from the occlusion of any of five vessels: vertebral, posterior inferior cerebellar, superior, middle or inferior lateral medullary arteries. Associated clinical features on the side of the lesion follow:

- Impaired pain and temperature sensation over half the face.
  Structure affected: nucleus and tract of trigeminal nerve.
- Limb ataxia, falling towards the side of the lesion.
  Structure affected: cerebellar hemisphere.
- Nystagmus, vertigo, nausea and vomiting.
  Structure affected: vestibular nucleus.
- Horner's syndrome.
  Structure affected: descending sympathetic tract.
- Paralysis of palatal and laryngeal muscles.
  Structure affected: fibres of IX and X nerves.
- Loss of taste (ageusia).
  Structure affected: nucleus and tractus solitarius.

Clinical features on the side opposite the lesion are impaired pain and temperature sense over half of the body; the structure affected is the spinothalamic tract.

9.15 (a) F (b) F (c) F (d) T (e) T
The normal volume of CSF in the subarachnoid space is 150 ml, and the rate of production is 550 ml/day. Approximately 50–70% is actively secreted by the choroid of the III, IV and lateral ventricles, the remainder being produced by ependymal cells lining the ventricles. CSF flows from the ventricles to the subarachnoid space *via* the foramina of Magendie and Luschka, and is reabsorbed by the arachnoid villi into cerebral blood vessels. The biochemical composition of CSF differs from that of plasma: in the CSF the sodium, potassium and calcium concentrations are lower, as is the pH (7.31–7.34). CSF glucose is typically 60–80% of the plasma glucose concentration. Concentrations of bicarbonate, chloride and magnesium are all higher in the CSF. Lumbar CSF pressure is normally 7–18 cmH_2O. CSF protein content is 0.2–0.5 g/l. Normal CSF leukocyte count is 0–3 cells/mm^3, 60–70% of which are lymphocytes. There are no neutrophils in a normal CSF sample. Levels of all immunoglobulins are lower in the CSF than in the plasma.

9.16 (a) T (b) T (c) F (d) F (e) F
The neuronal cell body (perikaryon) bears numerous processes (neurites). Neurites which conduct impulses towards the cell body are called dendrites, while those which conduct impulses away from the cell body are axons. Neurons may be classified according to the number of neurites, into unipolar, bipolar and multipolar neurons. Alternatively, they can be classified according to size: Golgi type I neurons have long axons (peripheral nerve fibres, Purkinje cells of cerebellar cortex and fibres of the long tracts); Golgi type II neurons have a short axon – these are more common than Golgi type I neurons.

The cell cytoplasm contains a nucleus, mitochondria, microtubules, lysosomes, centrioles, Golgi apparatus, lipofuscin, melanin, glycogen and lipid. The darkly staining Nissl substance, located in the cell body except at the region of the axon hillock, is composed of rough endoplasmic reticulum. The Golgi apparatus is important for the synthesis of synaptic vesicles at axon terminals; neurotransmitters are synthesized locally in the axon terminal.

9.17 (a) F (b) F (c) F (d) F (e) T
(See answer 9.18)

9.18 (a) T (b) F (c) F (d) T (e) T
The nerve cell membrane is polarized at rest, with a resting potential of –70mV, positive charges lined along the outside of the cell and negative charges on the inside. If a stimulus reaches threshold intensity an action potential is produced, regardless of the strength of that

stimulus above the threshold required, i.e. an all-or-none response. During depolarization, voltage-gated sodium channels open, resulting in influx of Na^+ and efflux of K^+, transiently reversing the polarity of the cell membrane. Increased chloride conductance of the axon is a feature of post-synaptic inhibition. During the refractory period (approximately 1 ms) a stimulus, no matter how strong, cannot excite the nerve: this depends on the speed of repolarization in that segment of cell membrane. The action potential moves along the axon at a constant amplitude and velocity.

The conduction velocity is up to 50 times more rapid in myelinated fibres as depolarization jumps from one node of Ranvier to the next along the axon (saltatory conduction). The speed of conduction also increases with increase in fibre diameter. A decrease in extracellular calcium ion concentration increases the excitability of both nerve and muscle cells by reducing the threshold required to initiate an action potential. In contrast, an increase in the extracellular calcium concentration decreases excitability by stabilizing the cell membrane.

9.19 (a) F (b) F (c) F (d) T (e) T

Table 9.1 Neurotransmitters in the central nervous system

Neurotransmitter	Receptor
Principal systems	
Acetylcholine	Nicotinic and muscarinic (M_1–M_5)
Adrenaline and noradrenaline	α and β
Dopamine	D_{1-5}
Serotonin	5-HT_{1-4}
Histamine	H_{1-3}
Excitatory amino acids	
Glutamate	Metabotropic and ionotropic
Aspartate	
Inhibitory amino acids	
Gamma-aminobutyric acid	$GABA_A$ and $GABA_B$
Glycine	
Tachykinins	
Substance P	NK_1
Neurokinins A and B	NK_2, NK_3
Opioid peptides	
Encephalins	μ, κ and δ
met-encephalin	
leu-encephalin	
endorphins	

5-Hydroxytryptophan is formed from the hydroxylation of tryptophan, and is decarboxylated to form 5-hydroxytryptamine (serotonin, 5-HT).

9.20 (a) F (b) T (c) F (d) F (e) F

ACh is synthesized in the presynaptic terminal from acetyl-coenzyme A (acetyl-CoA) and choline, catalysed by choline acetyltransferase. ACh is rapidly removed from the synaptic cleft by hydrolysis to choline and acetate, catalysed by the enzyme acetylcholinesterase. There is active reuptake of choline into the presynaptic terminals of cholinergic neurons.

Dopamine is formed by the hydroxylation and decarboxylation of the amino acid tyrosine, catalysed by the enzymes tyrosine hydroxylase and dopa decarboxylase. There is active reuptake of dopamine into presynaptic neurons via a Na^+/Cl^--dependent transporter.

Noradrenaline is synthesized by the hydroxylation of dopamine, catalysed by dopamine decarboxylase. There is active reuptake into the presynaptic terminal where the free catecholamine is oxidized by monoamine oxidase, located on the outer surface of the mitochondria in the presynaptic terminals. Adrenaline is formed by methylation of noradrenaline.

Serotonin (5-hydroxytryptamine, 5-HT) is synthesized from the amino acid tryptophan, catalysed by the enzymes tryptophan carboxylase and decarboxylase. Released serotonin is reabsorbed by active reuptake, and inactivated by monoamine oxidase.

With the exception of ACh, reuptake of all the above neurotransmitters is *via* a Na^+/Cl^--dependent transporter. A similar transport mechanism is responsible for reuptake of gamma-aminobutyric acid (GABA), glycine and choline. The reuptake transporter for glutamate is a Na^+-co-transport/K^+-countertransport mechanism, which is Cl^--independent.

9.21 (a) F (b) T (c) F (d) T (e) T

There are two types of acetylcholine receptor, based on their sensitivity to muscarine (an alkaloid responsible for the toxicity of some fungi) and nicotine.

Muscarinic receptors are located at postganglionic parasympathetic synapses and can be selectively blocked by atropine. Five types of cholinergic muscarinic receptor have been identified, designated M1–M5: M1 receptors are located in the brain, M2 receptors in the heart, M4 in the pancreas and M2 and M4 in smooth muscle. M3 and M5 have not been fully characterized. The heart receives parasympathetic cholinergic fibres from the vagus, which has a negative chronotropic effect mediated via the M2 receptor.

Nicotinic receptors are located at all autonomic ganglia and in the adrenal medulla, and can be blocked selectively by hexamethonium. The acetylcholine receptors at the neuromuscular junction are also nicotinic and are blocked by tubocurarine but not hexamethonium.

9.22 (a) T (b) T (c) T (d) T (e) T
(See Table 9.2)

9.23 (a) T (b) T (c) T (d) T (e) T
A reflex is defined as an involuntary response to a stimulus. A monosynaptic reflex arc consists of a receptor organ, an afferent neuron, an efferent neuron and an effector. In a spinal reflex arc, the receptor organ is located in the skin, in tendon or in muscle. Afferent type Ia fibres from the muscle spindle and type Ib fibres from Golgi tendon organ have cell bodies in the dorsal root ganglia and synapse with afferent neurons in the spinal cord.

When a reflex is evoked in a muscle (the protagonist), the muscles which oppose its action (the antagonists) relax. This is due to *reciprocal innervation*: the type Ia fibres from the muscle spindle have a collateral branch which passes to an inhibitory interneuron (Golgi bottle neuron): this synapses directly with the motor neuron innervating the antagonist muscle. Evoking a reflex on one side of the body causes the inverse effect on the limb of the other side. This is the *crossed extensor reflex*.

9.24 (a) F (b) F (c) T (d) F (e) F
Cell bodies of preganglionic neurons are located in the visceral efferent column of the spinal cord, or in the motor nuclei of the cranial nerves. Preganglionic neurons are mainly myelinated, slow conducting B fibres; the axons of postganglionic neurons are mainly unmyelinated C fibres. Autonomic neurons can be classified as cholinergic or noradrenergic according to the neurotransmitter released.

Cholinergic neurons are all preganglionic neurons, parasympathetic postganglionic neurons, sympathetic postganglionic neurons innervating sweat glands and sympathetic neurons mediating vasodilatation in skeletal muscle.

Noradrenergic neurons are the remaining postganglionic sympathetic neurons.

The parasympathetic outflow is divided into cranial and sacral portions: the cranial division supplies visceral structures in the head via oculomotor (III), facial (VII) and glossopharyngeal (XI) nerves, and structures in the thorax and upper abdomen *via* the vagus (X) nerve. The sacral outflow (S2–4) supplies the pelvic organs. Preganglionic parasympathetic fibres are long, ending on short postganglionic neurons. Sympathetic preganglionic neurons leave the spinal cord *via* the ventral roots of spinal nerves T1–L3. Most preganglionic fibres are short, synapsing with postganglionic neurons in the sympathetic chain.

Table 9.2 Erlanger/Gasser* and Lloyd/Hunt† classification of nerve fibres

Fibre type*		Number†	Myelinated	Diameter (μm)	Function
A	α	Ia	√	15	Motor to muscle spindle (annulospiral ending) [alpha motor neurons]
		Ib	√		Afferents from Golgi tendon organ
	β	II	√	8	Cutaneous touch and pressure afferents
	γ	—	√	5	Motor to muscle spindle (flower-spray ending) [gamma motor neurons]
	δ	III	√	< 3	Cutaneous pain and temperature afferents
B	—	—	√	3	Preganglionic sympathetic fibres
C	Dorsal root	IV	×	1	Cutaneous pain afferents
	Sympathetic	—	×		Postganglionic sympathetic fibres

9.25 (a) T (b) T (c) F (d) F (e) F
The most prominent component of the EEG in a resting adult with eyes closed is the **alpha rhythm** (8–12 cycles/s). This is most marked in the occipital area and is abolished when the eyes are opened. Alpha rhythm may be slowed in a number of toxic and metabolic diseases. The **beta rhythms** have faster frequencies (18–30 cycles/s) and are usually seen over the frontal regions and vertex. They may be abnormal over local, chronic lesions and may be enhanced by sedative drugs. **Theta waves** (4–8 cycles/s) are usually seen in the temporal regions in children, but are frequently associated with underlying disease in adults. **Delta waves** are large, slow (< 4 cycles/s) rhythms which are always abnormal in the alert adult. The EEG can be of diagnostic help in a number of conditions which have characteristic EEG abnormalities.

Petit-mal epilepsy shows a typical 3-Hz spike wave pattern. The EEG in CJD and subacute sclerosing panencephalitis shows periodic sharp waves. The recently described variant of CJD (nvCJD) does not exhibit these typical EEG features. Lateral periodic slow waves are seen in herpes simplex encephalitis; **triphasic waves** are a feature of some forms of metabolic encephalopathy. Periodic lateralized epileptiform discharges (PLEDS) may be seen over areas of acute hemispheric pathology (haematoma, abscess or rapidly expanding tumour). Non-specific focal slow waves occur over areas of haemorrhage, infarction or tumour.

FURTHER READING

Ganong, W.F. (1995) *Review of Medical Physiology*, 17th edn, Appleton & Lange, East Norwalk.

Moore, K.L. (1992) *Clinically Oriented Anatomy*, 3rd edn, Williams and Wilkins, Baltimore.

Rang, H.P. and Dale, M.M. (1995) *Pharmacology*, 3rd edn, Churchill Livingston, Edinburgh.

Snell, R.S. (1992) *Clinical Neuroanatomy for Medical Students*, 3rd edn, Little, Brown and Co., Boston.

10 Statistics and epidemiology

QUESTIONS

10.1 In a normal or Gaussian distribution:

(a) the mean, median and mode coincide.
(b) 95% of observations lie between the mean ±2 standard deviations ($\bar{x} \pm$ 2s.d.).
(c) 25% of observations lie between the mean +1 standard deviation ($\bar{x} +$ 1s.d.).
(d) data should be $\log_{10}$ transformed before analysis.
(e) the 95% confidence interval may be calculated as the product of 1.96 and the standard deviation in populations of greater than $n = 30$.

10.2 In the following study using prostate-specific antigen (PSA) to identify prostate cancer in males over 70 years old the following results were obtained:

PSA	**No prostate cancer**	**Prostate cancer**
Below 10 ng/ml	**440**	**8**
Above 10 ng/ml	**10**	**42**

The following statements are correct:

(a) the sensitivity of the test is 98%.
(b) there were 16% false-negatives.
(c) the predictive value of a positive test (PSA > 10 ng/ml) in diagnosing prostate cancer is 81%.
(d) there were 2% false-positives.
(e) the predictive value of a negative test (PSA < 10 ng/ml) is 98%.

10.3 Type II or β error is likely to occur in the interpretation of a clinical trial:

(a) if a sample size is small.
(b) if a large number of variables are tested using a *t*-test.
(c) if there is variability of patient response to the treatment.
(d) if 95% confidence intervals are used to compare the difference between treatments.
(e) if the significance value for the major endpoint is $P < 0.001$.

10.4 Meta-analysis of randomized controlled trials:

(a) is usually performed when individual trials are too small to give reliable answers.
(b) should only include published 'peer-reviewed' studies.
(c) provides a more stable estimate of the effect of treatment than individual trials.
(d) should exclude trials in which patient selection is not randomized.
(e) provides conclusions which make the performance of further controlled trials unnecessary.

10.5 In a clinical trial of a new drug treatment:

(a) allocation of treatment to each patient should be determined by disease severity.
(b) baseline variables in patients allocated to different treatment groups are reduced by randomized allocation.
(c) the null hypothesis is rejected if there are significant differences in response in randomly allocated treatment groups.
(d) patients receiving placebo treatment may improve.
(e) random allocation of treatment eliminates assessment bias.

10.6 A sample contains the values 2, 2, 2, 2, 2, 4, 5, 5, 6, 7:

(a) the mean is 3.7.
(b) the median is 4.
(c) the distribution is normal.
(d) the mode is 2.
(e) the standard deviation is $\sqrt{\frac{\text{mean}}{n}}$.

10.7 The standard deviation of a group of observations:

(a) is the square root of the variance of the group.
(b) is a measure of the scatter of the observations around their mean.
(c) is a valid statistical parameter only if the observations recorded have a normal (Gaussian) distribution.
(d) is numerically higher than the standard error of the mean for the group.
(e) may be used as a basis for the calculation of chi-squared.

10.8 Nonparametric methods of statistical analysis include:

(a) Mann–Whitney *U* test.
(b) Kruskall–Wallis analysis of variance.

(c) the paired *t*-test.
(d) Kendal's rank correlation test.
(e) the sign test.

10.9 A report of a clinical trial of a new anti-hypertensive drug states: 'In a comparison between the new drug and a placebo, a higher proportion of patients taking the new drug had a fall in diastolic blood pressure of more than 5 mmHg ($P < 0.05$)'. It can be inferred that:
(a) the trial was a randomized double-blind placebo controlled study.
(b) a placebo response is likely to have occurred in 5% of patients.
(c) the 95% confidence intervals of the change in blood pressure would be more useful than a *P* value.
(d) blood pressure was measured using a random zero sphygmomanometer.
(e) the result should be regarded as reaching conventional levels of statistical significance.

10.10 The following statements are correct:
(a) a correlation coefficient (r) can range from −1 to +1.
(b) the significance of a correlation coefficient can be determined from the '*t*' distribution.
(c) the variance of a normal distribution can be calculated from the standard deviation (s.d.).
(d) a *P* value of 0.1 for the difference between two means is more significant than one of 0.01.
(e) the standard error of the mean (s.e.m.) can be calculated as the standard deviation divided by the mean (s.d./$\overline{x}$).

10.11 Ninety-five percent confidence intervals (c.i.'s):
(a) comparing two populations indicate no difference if zero lies within them.
(b) are a test of the null hypothesis.
(c) indicate the range in which there is a 95% chance of the true population mean lying.
(d) can be calculated for non-parametric data.
(e) are useful when comparing data with another population.

10.12 Relative risk
(a) is a useful measure of the association between a disease and a risk factor.
(b) is defined as the incidence rate of disease in an exposed group.
(c) is best assessed in retrospective case control studies.

(d) of 2 indicates a doubling of risk between the groups.
(e) is equivalent to an odds ratio.

10.13 In a study of the incidence of coronary heart disease (CHD) in smokers over 60 years the following results were obtained:

		CHD	
		Yes	**No**
Smoker	**Yes**	**500**	**2000**
	No	**100**	**4900**

The following statements are correct:
(a) smokers have a higher incidence than non-smokers of CHD.
(b) the relative risk for coronary artery disease in smokers compared to non-smokers is 5.
(c) the odds ratio for smokers compared to non-smokers is 12.25.
(d) confidence limits for the odds ratio cannot be calculated.
(e) chi-squared is an appropriate test of significance.

10.14 In a clinical trial of a new drug, the following results were obtained:

	Drug	Placebo
No. of patients improved	**36**	**29**
No. of patients not improved	**14**	**21**

The following statements are correct:
(a) 28% of patients receiving the new drug improved.
(b) if a test of significance were required, computation of linear regression would be appropriate.
(c) the data could be evaluated by calculating chi-squared.
(d) the data could be evaluated by calculating Student's *t*.
(e) if the probability that the difference between the drug and placebo is due to chance is 0.1, the drug can be introduced into clinical practice.

10.15 Evidence-based medicine:
(a) is restricted to randomized placebo-controlled trials.
(b) may involve a health economics assessment.
(c) is a method for rationing resources in a health care system.
(d) combines clinical expertise and external evidence.
(e) relies only on objective measurements of disease outcomes.

10.16 Life table analysis:
(a) can only be used to study mortality risk factors in a population.
(b) uses prevalence data from the population.

(c) can be used to calculate relative risk.
(d) can be adjusted to allow for covariables.
(e) from two groups can be compared by calculation of a chi-squared statistic.

10.17 When comparing two independent methods of clinical measurement:
(a) a paired *t*-test is a suitable method of analysis.
(b) a regression line of the results for the two methods should have a gradient of 5.
(c) a regression line of the results for the two methods should have an intercept of 0.
(d) if the difference between the measurement increases with the averages of the two measurements, the methods are comparable.
(e) the chi-squared test will test how closely they agree.

10.18 When comparing two groups of data:
(a) ordinal data is best tested by a parametric test.
(b) dichotomous data is best tested by a chi-squared test.
(c) very small samples ($n < 5$ in each group) should be tested using a Mann–Whitney *U* test.
(d) a two sample *t*-test is suitable for interval data which is not normally distributed.
(e) nominal data can be tested by Fisher's exact test.

10.19 If a characteristic is normally distributed in a population:
(a) this implies that most of the population are normal individuals.
(b) there will be equal numbers who have more or less of the characteristic than the mean.
(c) 20% of individuals will be beyond two standard deviations from the mean.
(d) the median value will be less than the mean.
(e) the modal value will be identical with the mean.

10.20 The peak expiratory flow rates (PEFRs) of a group of 15-year old boys are normally distributed with a mean of 400 l/min and a standard deviation of 50 l/min. It follows that:
(a) about 70% of the boys have PEFRs between 300 and 500 l/min.
(b) 50% of the boys have a PEFR above 400 l/min.
(c) the boys have healthy lungs.
(d) about 5% of the boys have PEFRs below 300 l/min.
(e) all the PEFRs must be less than 500 l/min.

10.21 When calculating the size of a sample required for a study comparing a new drug to placebo:

(a) it is necessary to define the most important endpoint for the study.
(b) an estimate of the standard deviation of the parameter of interest is required.
(c) maximum power is usually achieved by having equal numbers in both groups.
(d) only variables which are continuous can be used.
(e) the probability of rejecting the null hypothesis when it is false is termed the power.

10.22 The following statements regarding mortality rates are correct:

(a) crude mortality rates are calculated only from death certificate data.
(b) the standardized mortality ratio (SMR) is the expected number of deaths divided by observed number of deaths for a specified group.
(c) they are usually standardized for age and sex.
(d) in males over the age of 15 years age-specific death rates increase by 10–20% for each subsequent 5-year period.
(e) they provide important information about the changing pattern of disease in society.

10.23 In an epidemiological study of the effect of diet on coronary artery disease:

(a) the number of coronary events is a relevant outcome variable.
(b) a calculation of sample size is not important.
(c) cigarette smoking may be a confounding variable.
(d) a pilot study may be valuable.
(e) dietary intakes can be accurately measured by postal questionnaire.

10.24 A coefficient of correlation:

(a) must be between −1 and +1.
(b) can only be determined in normally distributed data.
(c) measures the size of change of one variable compared to another.
(d) of 0.95 is usually statistically significant.
(e) of 0.95 usually indicates causation between the two factors.

10.25 Analysis of variance (ANOVA):
(a) is a method of comparing three or more groups.
(b) assumes similar variances in each group.
(c) uses the *t* distribution for significance testing.
(d) requires equal numbers in each group.
(e) gives a probability value (*P*) for each comparison of the mean of each group.

ANSWERS

10.1 (a) T (b) T (c) F (d) F (e) F
The normal or Gaussian (Gauss 1777–1855) distribution is the most important frequency distribution in statistics. The properties of a normal distribution are:

1. symmetrical about the mean, so that the mean, median and mode coincide;
2. 68% of observations lie within 1 s.d. (σ) of the mean ($\overline{x}$) $\pm$ 1 s.d.,
   95% lie between $\overline{x} \pm 2$ s.d.,
   99.7% lie between $\overline{x} \pm 3$ s.d.;
3. because of this symmetry, about 34% of observations lie between $\overline{x}$ and $\overline{x}$ + 1 s.d.

Data from a normal distribution is suitable for parametric tests without prior transformation. Observations which do not conform to a normal distribution may be log-normally distributed and can be transformed to a normal distribution by converting values to $\log_{10}$, Counts of events (e.g. bacterial colonies, radioactive counts) may follow a Poisson distribution and may be suitably transformed by taking the square root value.

The 95% confidence interval gives information about the range of values within which the true population is likely to lie. The 95% confidence intervals are calculated as the mean ± 1.96 times the standard error of the mean (s.e.m.) for populations of greater than 30. For smaller populations the appropriate value of *t* can be taken from appropriate tables such that the 95% confidence levels are calculated as ($\overline{x}$ – (*t* × s.e.m.)) – ($\overline{x}$ + (*t* × s.e.m.), where *t* is taken for the appropriate degrees of freedom associated with a confidence interval of 95% 100(1-α)%, i.e. 0.05.

10.2 (a) F (b) T (c) T (d) T (e) T
The sensitivity of a test = $\dfrac{\text{number tested positive}}{\text{total with condition}}$
i.e. 42/50 × 100 = 84% and 16% false-positives.

$$\text{The specificity of a test} = \frac{\text{number tested negative}}{\text{total without the condition}}$$

i.e. 440/450 × 100 = 98% and 2% false-positives.

The predictive value of a negative test is 440/448 × 100 = 98.2%.

The predictive value of a positive test is 42/52 × 100 = 81%.

10.3 (a) T (b) F (c) T (d) F (e) F

Type I error or α error is wrongly rejecting the null hypothesis, e.g. interpretation of $P < 0.05$ as being significant when it is not.

Type II error or β error is accepting the null hypothesis when it is invalid, e.g. when two treatments are compared and no significant difference ($P > 0.05$) is noted, assuming there is no difference between them when there is in fact a difference.

Both types of error are more likely to occur when small samples are used. Type I error is more likely to occur when multiple *t*-tests are performed. Type II errors are often related to variability of response to treatment and this form of misinterpretation is reduced by the use of confidence intervals. Narrow 95% confidence intervals allow more certain conclusions to be drawn on data.

10.4 (a) T (b) F (c) T (d) T (e) F

Meta-analysis of randomized controlled trials is usually performed when individually the trials are too small to five reliable answers. There are a number of reasons for performing meta-analysis, which include:

1. to examine variability between trials;
2. to perform subgroup analysis;
3. to identify the need for major trials;
4. to obtain a more stable estimate of the effect of treatment.

Only randomized controlled trials should be included in such analysis, but if only published studies (which tend to be positive) are used this will introduce bias. If unpublished but properly controlled studies are available they should be used in the analysis. It is important that patient selection and outcomes are comparable in the studies. Meta-analysis does not take the place of properly controlled large studies to answer important questions, but may help in the appropriate design of such trials.

10.5 (a) F (b) T (c) T (d) T (e) F

When comparing a new drug to placebo or current best treatment the best method is a randomized double-blind study. Patients should be unselected and, on entry into the study, randomly allocated to the new drug or the placebo treatment. This can be achieved from a random number table and allocating even numbers to one treatment and odd numbers to the other. Random allocation then allows examination of the null hypothesis which is that there is no difference between the treatments. Significant differences between the two treatment groups allow the null hypothesis to be rejected. Baseline differences may occur in studies of small numbers of patients; the larger the groups the less likely there is to be a significant difference between the two groups. Random allocation does not affect assessment bias. This is eliminated by the treatments being blinded to patient and doctor. Patients receiving placebo may improve because of the natural history of their disease or, in some situations, because of the increased doctor input associated with clinical trials.

10.6 (a) T (b) F (c) F (d) T (e) F
The mean value is $\Sigma x/n = 37/10 = 3.7$.

The median value is the central value = 2.

The mode is the most commonly occurring value = 2.

This is not a normal distribution. It is skewed towards the left. These data may require a transformation before analysis.

The standard deviation is derived from the variance (s^2) of data.

$$s^2 = \frac{\Sigma(x-\overline{x})^2}{(n-1)}$$

The term $\Sigma(x-\overline{x})^2$ is often called the sum of squares. The standard deviation is $\sqrt{s^2}$.

10.7 (a) T (b) T (c) T (d) T (e) F
The variance (s^2) of a group of observations is calculated as follows:

$$s^2 = \frac{\Sigma(x-\overline{x})^2}{(n-1)}$$

The standard deviation (s.d.) is the square root of the variance:

$$\text{s.d.} = \sqrt{s^2}.$$

The s.d. is an estimate of expected variation from the mean and assumes the observations come from a normal distribution. Data which is not normally distributed will often yield a very large s.d. which may be greater than the mean.

The standard error of the mean (s.e.m.) is calculated as:

$$\text{s.e.m.} = \sqrt{s^2/n} = \text{s.d.}/\sqrt{n}$$

i.e. standard deviation/square root of the number in the study group.

The s.e.m. is always less than the s.d., which is not used in the calculation of chi-squared.

10.8 (a) T (b) T (c) F (d) T (e) T
Parametric tests assume a normal distribution and should be applied to the analysis of data which reasonably conforms to this. Parametric tests include tests based on Student's *t*-distribution and least squares regression. Parametric tests comparing two populations also assume that the variances in the two groups are the same.

Nonparametric tests do not assume any particular distribution. Ordinal data is particularly well suited to nonparametric tests. Examples include Mann–Whitney *U* test, Wilcoxon matched pairs test, sign test and Kruskal–Wallis nonparametric analysis of variance for multiple groups (three or more).

Correlation can be calculated from parametric data from the product moment correlation for normally distributed interval data and the Spearman or Kendall's rank correlation coefficient for data not normally distributed.

All nonparametric tests depend on ranking of data. The choice between parametric and nonparametric tests depends on the study performed and should be suited to the problem, bearing in mind assumptions regarding distribution and variances of the data.

10.9 (a) F (b) F (c) T (d) F (e) T
The design of the trial cannot be inferred from the above statement. Such a trial should be randomized, double-blind and placebo-controlled. The report indicates that the effect of the drug on diastolic blood pressure is unlikely to be because of chance ($P < 0.05$) and the null hypothesis can be rejected. If the null hypothesis is true (i.e. no difference), this will be wrong on less than one occasion in 20. The conventional level of statistical significance is 5% ($P = 0.05$). This is a good guideline for significance but should not be taken as an absolute demarcation. The magnitude of the difference is better expressed as the 95% confidence interval of the difference in diastolic blood pressure. The *P* value only indicates a difference, while confidence intervals tell us by how much.

10.10 (a) T (b) T (c) T (d) F (e) F
This question addresses a number of statistical tests.

Coefficient of correlation (r) can be from -1 to $+1$. The closer r is to -1 or $+1$, the more likely it is to be a significant correlation and the probability of significance depends on the degrees of freedom. This can be determined from the *t*-distribution. An r value of zero indicates no correlation.

The variance is the square of the standard deviation.

As P values decrease the more significant the difference between groups and the more confidently the null hypothesis can be rejected. P values do not give an indication of the magnitude of any difference. Confidence intervals are more valuable to indicate this.

The standard error of the mean (s.e.m.) is the standard deviation divided by the square root of the total (n).

10.11 (a) T (b) F (c) T (d) T (e) T

In a normal distribution of a large population (>30), 95% confidence intervals (c.i.) can be calculated as ± 1.96 times the standard error of the mean. This means there is a 95% chance that the true population mean will lie within the range of values.

Ninety-five per cent c.i. can be calculated for nonparametric or interval data but this uses a different method than $1.96 \times$ s.e.m.

When comparing the effects of two treatments (e.g. active drug and placebo or two populations) 95% c.i. indicate the size of any effect rather than just indicating if there was an effect, as in significance testing. There is a close relationship between the use of c.i. and the two-sided hypothesis test.

When comparing two groups, if zero difference lies within the 95% c.i. this indicates no effect.

10.12 (a) T (b) F (c) F (d) T (e) F

Relative risk may be determined in prospective and retrospective studies and is a useful measure of the strength of association between disease and a risk factor. In a prospective study of a population, participants are selected without reference to the presence or absence of disease. After excluding prevalence cases the population is followed over time. The number of new cases occurring thereafter is divided by the population at risk, giving an incidence rate. The relative risk is calculated as:

$$\text{relative risk} = \frac{\text{incidence rate of disease in an exposed group}}{\text{incidence rate of disease in an unexposed group}}$$

		Cases	Non-cases
Risk factor	Yes	A	B
	No	C	D

In contrast, an odds ratio is the ratio of the odds of disease to non-disease in those with a risk factor, divided by the odds of disease to non-disease in those with no risk factor. The ratios are illustrated in the 2×2 table above.

$$\text{Relative risk} = \frac{A/(A + B)}{C/(C + D)}$$

$$\text{Odds ratio} = \frac{A/B}{C/D}$$

10.13 (a) T (b) F (c) T (d) F (e) T
This is a 2 × 2 table from which relative risk and odds ratio can be calculated. Smokers have a higher incidence of CHD (0.2 or 20%) compared to an incidence of 0.02 or 2% in non-smokers.

$$\text{Relative risk} = \frac{500/2500}{100/5000}$$
$$= 0.2/0.02$$
$$= 10.$$

$$\text{Odds ratio (OR)} = \frac{500/2000}{100/4900}$$
$$= 0.0025/0.0204$$
$$= 12.25.$$

Confidence intervals can be calculated from the standard error of the natural log (ln) of the odds ratio:

$$\text{s.e. (ln OR)} = (1/a + 1/b + 1/c + 1/d)^{1/2}.$$

$$\text{and 95\% c.i.} = \ln \text{OR} \pm 1.96\,(1/a + 1/b + 1/c + 1/d)^{1/2}.$$

10.14 (a) F (b) F (c) T (d) F (e) F
This is a straightforward 2 × 2 table with a dichotomous variable, improved or not improved. Chi-squared is the most appropriate method of analysis. The parametric *t*-test is appropriate for the comparison of two mean values from normally distributed parameters. Linear regression also relies on analysis of a continuous variable and examines the relationship of $y = mx + c$ and is not appropriate to analyse this data.

Thirty-six of fifty patients receiving the drug improved, i.e. 72%, and 29 of 50 who had placebo improved, i.e. 58%. A probability of 0.1 is not significant. Showing statistical significance in an efficiency endpoint is not sufficient justification for inclusion of a drug into clinical practice. Adverse events, the magnitude of improvement, comparison to conventional treatment and health economics appraisal, amongst others, are important in such an assessment.

10.15 (a) F (b) T (c) F (d) T (e) F

'Evidence-based medicine is the conscientious, explicit and judicious use of current best evidence in making decisions about care of individual patients. This means integrating individual clinical expertise with the best available external evidence'. (*BMJ* 1996, **812**, 71–2).

Clinical expertise involves proficiency and judgement gained by clinicians with time and the compassionate application of knowledge to individuals. Current best evidence comes form many sources, including randomized controlled trials, meta-analysis, national expert guidelines (e.g. hypertension and asthma), patient-orientated studies and health economic assessment.

Evidence-based medicine is not 'cook-book' medicine, a method for cost-cutting, and does not solely rely on randomized controlled trials.

10.16 (a) F (b) F (c) T (d) T (e) T

Life table analysis is used in various contexts to follow a population until certain endpoints occur. Death is a suitable endpoint but development of disease or disability are also appropriate. For example, the mortality rates in groups of smokers and non-smokers could be collected over a period of time and survival plotted as a function of time. The development of retinopathy in diabetics, or the time from treatment of multiple sclerosis patients treated with α interferon or placebo to next relapse would also be suitable for life table analysis. These incidence data are best collected prospectively.

Life tables from two groups can be compared by calculating a chi-squared statistic (Mantel–Haenszel procedure or log rank method). Relative risk can also be calculated from such data.

Mathematical models can be applied to life table data to adjust for confounding variables (covariables). An example of this is the Cox proportional hazards model.

10.17 (a) F (b) F (c) T (d) F (e) F

The comparison of two independent methods of measurement can be done by plotting a scatter diagram. If two methods are comparable the regression line should go through zero and the gradient should be 1 (i.e. $y = 1x + 0$ or $y = x$). This is not the best way to plot the data as all the points lie roughly along the line of equality. A plot of the average for each pair against the difference should be a horizontal line and all points be within the 95% limits of agreement (Bland and

Altman plot). If the difference increases with the subject mean the methods are not comparable. A paired test or chi-squared test are not suitable methods for comparison.

10.18 (a) F (b) T (c) F (d) F (e) T
There are basically three types of measurement scales:

1. **interval scale** – the size of the difference between two values has a consistent meaning, e.g. height, temperature;
2. **ordinal scale** – observations are ordered but differences on the scale may not have the same meaning, e.g. depression scores, Borg score;
3. **nominal scale** – qualitative or categorical variables where individuals are grouped but not ordered, e.g. hair colour. Dichotomous scales are nominal scales with only two categories.

The type of data influences the type of statistical test as shown below:

Scale	**Method**
Interval	normal distribution, *t*-test non-normal distribution, Mann–Whitney *U* test
Ordinal	Mann–Whitney *U* test
Nominal	Chi-squared test Fisher's exact test

Very small samples of interval data are probably best analysed by a *t*-test.

10.19 (a) F (b) T (c) F (d) F (e) T
The normal or Gaussian distribution is a probability distribution and implies nothing about the health or normality of the individuals. The mean is a measure of central tendency and there are equal numbers either side of the mean. Two standard deviations account for 95% of observations, so only 5% of individuals will go beyond two standard deviations either side of the mean. In a normal distribution the mean, median and mode coincide.

10.20 (a) F (b) T (c) F (d) F (e) F
In a normal distribution a range of 1.96 (approximately two) standard deviations on either side of the mean will cover 95% of the area under

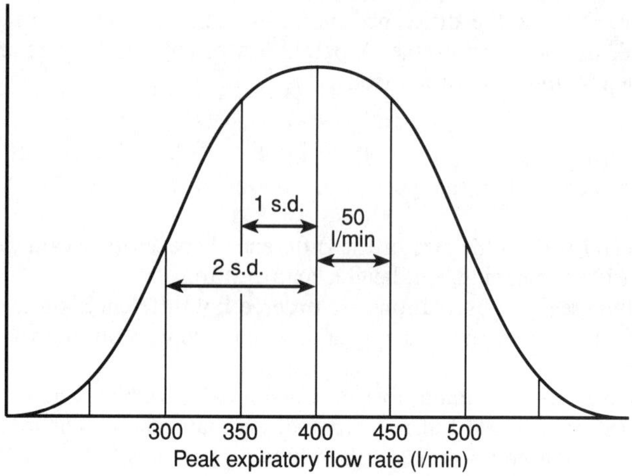

Figure 10.1 Normal distribution.

the curve. Of the sample, 2.5% will lie in the tail. Three standard deviations on either side of the mean will cover 99.7% of the area (Figure 3.1).

10.21 (a) T (b) T (c) T (d) F (e) T
Sample sizes can be calculated for population studies, clinical trials and most other forms of studies. Binary, ordered categorical and continuous variables can be used. It is very important before commencing clinical trial to determine which variable will be the primary endpoint, what magnitude of difference is clinically relevant and have an estimate of the standard deviation (s.d.). From these data and statistical significance (α), usually $P = 0.05$, the probability of rejecting the null hypothesis when it is false can be determined and is called the power (1 – β). With the expected mean difference/s.d. and a decision of significance and power, a sample size can be calculated.

Maximum power is achieved by having equal groups, but unequal group size can be used.

10.22 (a) F (b) T (c) T (d) F (e) T
Mortality rates are a very important source of information about the changing pattern of disease in a country. Most countries have a death certification system and data from this source can be combined with population census information to calculate a crude mortality rate.

$$\text{The crude mortality rate (deaths/1000/year)} = \frac{\text{deaths occurring over a 1-year period}}{\text{number in population at midpoint of year}}$$

Mortality rates are better expressed as age-specific death for males and females, and are usually started at 15–19 years, and increased in 5-year intervals. There is little change in the age-specific mortality rate between 15 and 34 years. After 45 years it approximately doubles over each 5-year period.

The standardized mortality ratio is a ratio of expected deaths in an age group (calculated from age-specific death rates) divided by the actual number of deaths in a specific group within that age group.

10.23 (a) T (b) F (c) T (d) T (e) F

The collection of data for epidemiological studies is crucial. The methods of obtaining data for studies should be very carefully thought through before commencing a study. The following are some important factors to be considered:

- defined objectives and outcome measures
- study population and sample size
- written protocol and tools (e.g. questionnaire)
- training of study staff
- pilot study
- likely response and adherence to the protocol
- allowance for confounding variables.

In the above suggested study coronary events are a relevant outcome measure and should be compared in groups with different diet, e.g. cholesterol intake, vitamin intake. Information on confounding variables such as cigarette smoking, family history and exercise should be collected. A pilot study is often very useful in determining potential problems and provides valuable data for calculation of sample size. Questionnaires are not an accurate way to assess diet and postal questionnaires usually have a poor response rate.

10.24 (a) T (b) F (c) F (d) T (e) F

Regression and correlation are often mixed up. Regression examines the nature of a relationship between two variables (i.e. how one changes against the other), while correlation tells us how close this relationship is. A coefficient of correlation can be calculated for parametric product moment correlation coefficient or ordinal data (Spearman's or Kendall's rank correlation coefficient).

A coefficient of correlation must lie between –1 and +1 and the higher the numerical value the more likely the correlation will be significant at the 0.05 level. This can be calculated from, for example, the *t*-distribution. Correlation does not indicate causation between the two variables.

10.25 (a) T (b) T (c) F (d) F (e) F

In studies where three or more groups are compared, the use of repeated *t*-tests for each pair of groups has disadvantages. The more groups (and therefore *t*-tests) the greater the probability of a significant difference when the null hypothesis is true (type I or α error). Analysis of variance (ANOVA) overcomes this by firstly calculating the common variance within groups. The variance of the total group (total sum of squares) and between groups variance can also be calculated. This allows the calculation of a variance ratio F (between groups mean square divided by within groups mean square). A probability value at the appropriate degrees of freedom can be found in a table of the F distribution.

ANOVA between groups assumes equal variances in each group but does not require groups to be of equal number.

Index

Page numbers in *italics* refer to questions; numbers in **bold** refer to figures and tables